body &soul

Dianne Wilson's experience as a fashion model, best selling author and speaker on the topics of Body & Soul have helped her live The Body & Soul Lifestyle to recover her shape and keep it after giving birth to four children including twins!

The cover of this book is a photograph of Dianne taken after she successfully lost 75 pounds, living The Body & Soul Lifestyle.

Dianne, alongside her husband Jonathan, are the Senior Pastors of Newport Church in Orange County, California, USA.

> Beloved, I pray that you may prosper in every way
> And [that your body] may keep well,
> Even as [I know] your soul keeps well and prospers.
> 3 John 1:2

With love
from Dianne xx

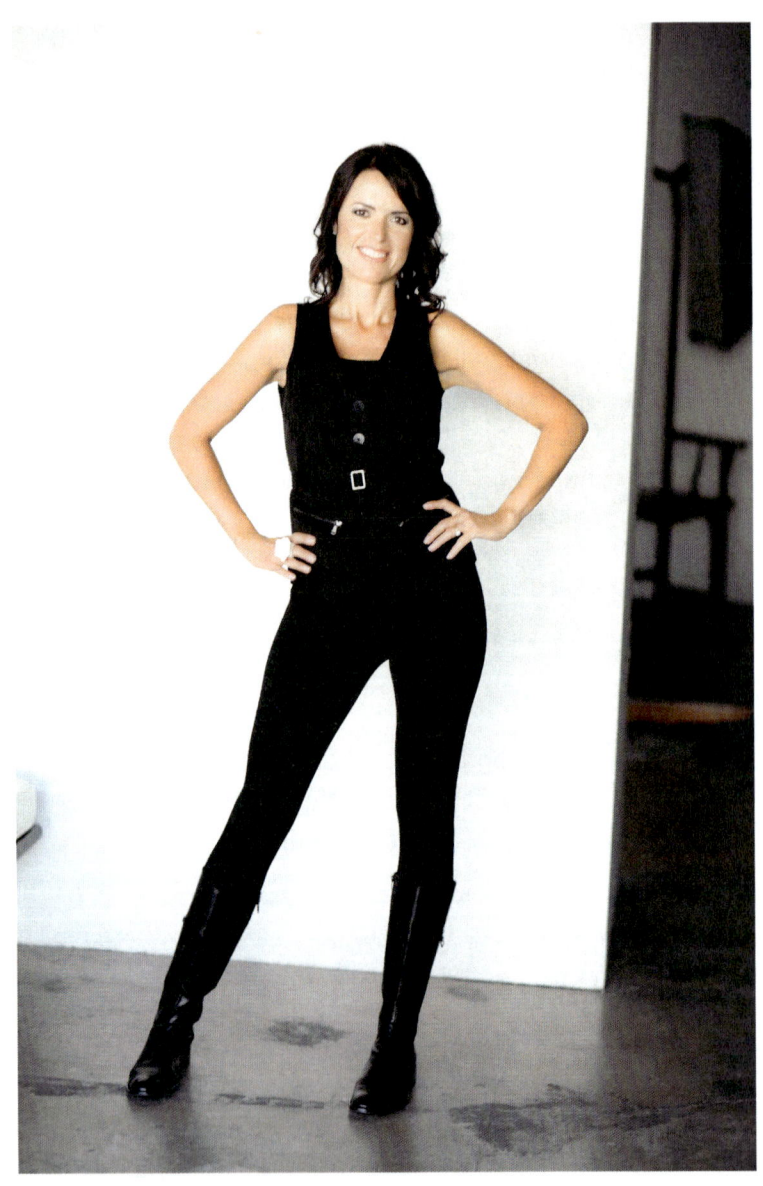

Welcome to a new beginning…

body & soul

The Lifestyle

Dianne Wilson

Body & Soul Published by Dianne Wilson

First published as Fat Free Forever! by Mandarin [Reed Books] 1996
First published as Fat Free Forever! by Random House Australia 1997
Reprinted 1998 [three times]; 1999; 2001
Random House Australia revised edition first published 2002

Photography: Nicole Caldwell: www.nicolecaldwell.com
Cover Graphics: Corey Meyers
Typeset in Newport Beach California
Printed in the USA

Author Contact Details:
Dianne Wilson
Newport Church
PO Box 9577 . Newport Beach . CA . 92657 . USA
Email: dianne.wilson@newportchurch.com
Tel: +1.949.706.2812

The author and the publisher of this book are not medically trained and are not licensed to give medical advice. Always consult your doctor before embarking on any weight loss course. The facts provided are based on extensive research up until the publishing date; however, the contents of products mentioned are subject to change by manufacturers from time to time and those contents may vary from those listed in this book.

Although a useful guide when shopping, information in this book is not an endorsement or recommendation of any product, manufacturer, company or individual. The author and publisher of this book cannot take responsibility for any injuries incurred by readers in performing any of the exercises outlined in this guide. As with any program of exercise, it should be undertaken with care and with individuals working at their own pace. Exercise guidelines have been provided to assist the reader. The author and the publisher recommend that a sound base of knowledge be developed by the user prior to embarking on any exercise program. The author and publisher disclaim any liability, damage or loss whatsoever arising directly or indirectly from the information contained in Body & Soul.

10 9 8 7 6 5 4 3 2 1

Foreword

Cardiovascular disease remains the largest single cause of death amongst Australians [and Americans]. This is true of many western countries. In addition, there are other large, often forgotten, non-lethal consequences such as time lost from work, hospitalization, and long-term symptoms as a result of cardiovascular disease.

Body & Soul is a very informative, easy to read and easy to follow piece of literature. It has great recipes sensibly listed under different food categories.

The book is enthusiastically written and I hope its readers will be contagiously affected by Dianne Wilson's optimistic style.

Finally, don't start changing things tomorrow – start now!

David W. Baron, FRACP Cardiologist
St. Vincent's Hospital Sydney, Australia

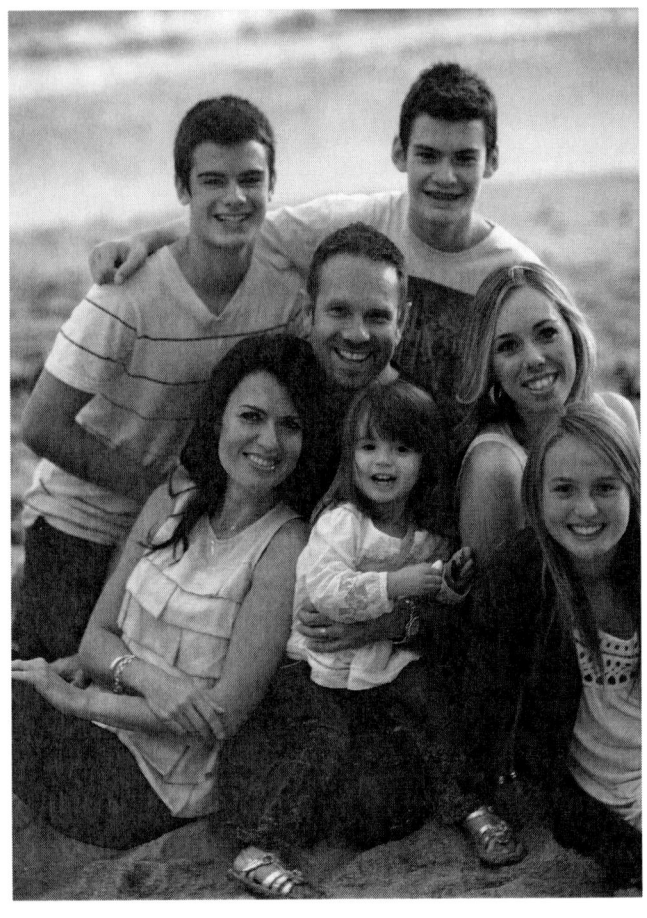

To my precious baby girl London Eternity,
It is only fitting that Mummy should dedicate
this book to you.
After all, if it wasn't for you, I wouldn't know if I had it in me
to get back in shape one more time!
We did it kiddo – you and me!
Ben and Beau, thank you for *Fat Free Forever!*
Beautiful Bella, thank you for *Back in Shape After Baby!*
Thank you London Eternity for
Body & Soul.

Thank you …

I am the most blessed woman in the whole wide world. I have the most wonderful family; I often wonder how that happened!

My spectacular husband Jonathan, Te Amo baby!

My stellar children – London Eternity, Bella Elena, Bentley Scott, Beaucara Calder, Rachel Claire and Joshua Christopher, you make motherhood my big time favorite focus!

My stunning family – Mum and Dad, and my sister Kathy; thank you for always teaching me to dream a bigger dream and that life's problems are really special opportunities for us to learn and grow through.

I am surrounded by some of the most magnificent team of people here in Newport that I have ever known; Wonder Women personified! There are more names than I can possibly list who are part of a deep ocean of love in my life.

Thank you, Nicole Caldwell, for making me look as beautiful as I feel.

Michelle Tolliver, the best personal trainer in the world. My friend and a true soul sister – thank you for believing in me, inspiring me, and for being my mirror so I could believe before I could see.

Thank you, Jesus, for true FREEDOM!

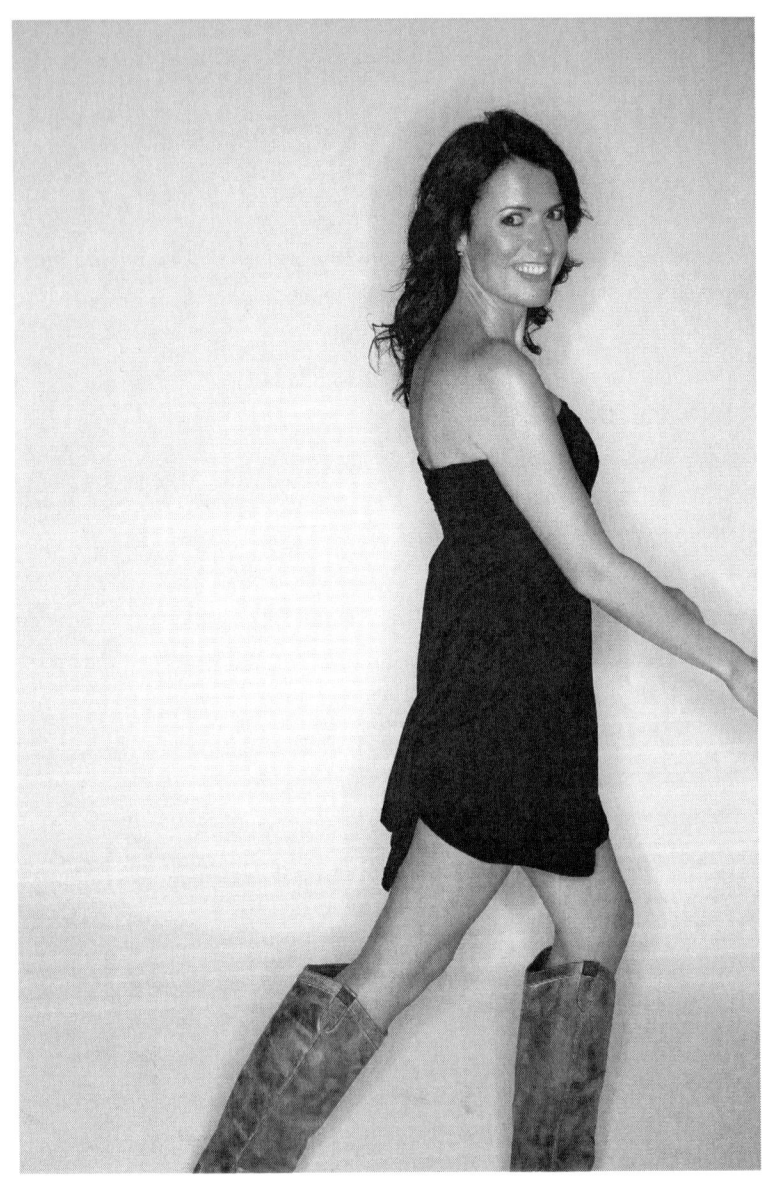

Let's go!

Contents

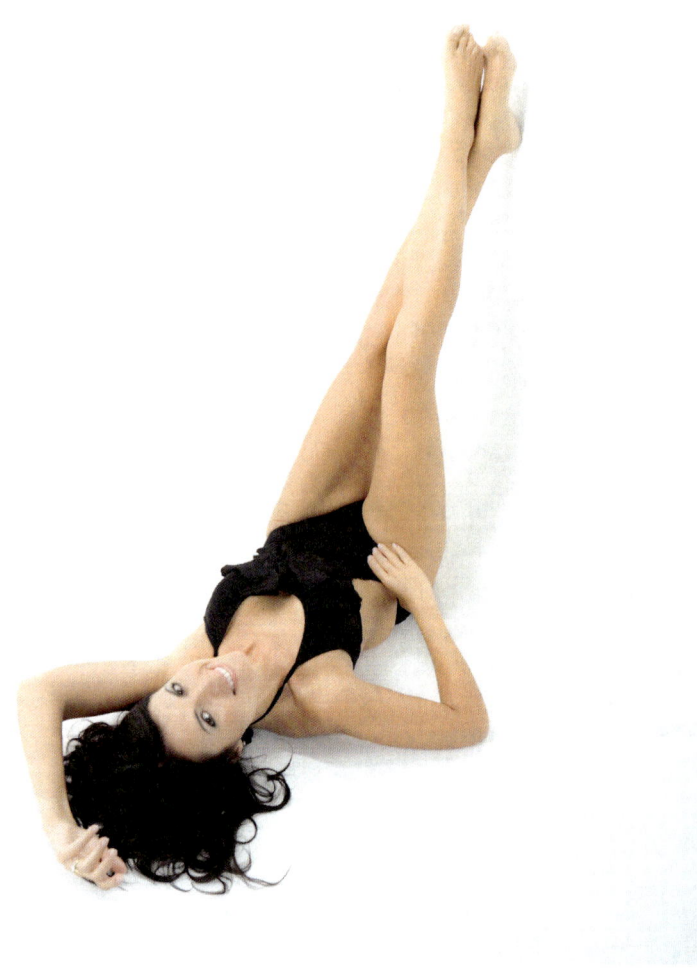

Hi

My Story

My account of something happening.

It's time to welcome the change coming soon into your life. What an exciting thought!

Life is full of choices and this is my story.

If you eat unhealthily, you will be unhealthy.

If you overload on starchy carbohydrates [cereal, bread, potato, rice and pasta], you will put on weight.

And if you starve yourself to be thin, you will gain even more weight [eventually].

I have done the lot, and believe me – it's true.

From my mid-teens to early twenties, I went through the whole 'yo-yo' dieting thing, along with most of the other girls I knew. I would starve myself for a week just to fit into a pair of tiny jeans. I also suffered greatly when I had to eat in front of people. I was so nervous.

One summer when I was away on holidays, I grazed on carrots and apples and drank only water for days on end.

> The greatest problem with not eating was that all I was doing was starving my muscle tissue and ruining my body shape.

I certainly was the skinniest girl on the beach that summer. Sure, I lost weight, but the less I ate, the more my poor body cried 'starvation', and clicked itself into a mode that was designed to store fat in times of ' famine' for protection. This made it nearly impossible to keep the weight off. I have learned that people are typically emotional eaters or emotional starvers. I was both — depending on the circumstances!

> If the enemy knows you live by your *feelings*
> he will *feed* you everything you *feel* like.
> Don't fall for it!

The greatest problem with not eating was that all I was doing was starving my muscle tissue and ruining my body shape. This is why emotional eaters usually head for the potato chips, buttered toast, peanut butter, hamburgers and chocolate. It takes a while for some people to realize that true comfort cannot come from a crinkle-cut anything. An instant 'high' soon converts to a long-term 'low'.

During all of this unintended craziness, though, I didn't know about or give a second thought to what this was doing to my body's metabolism.

When I was growing up, we always had non-fat milk and lots of fresh fruit in our house. We would arrive home each afternoon after school and Mum would hand my sister and me a carrot on our way through the front door. Lemonade was a special treat, as were chocolate biscuits.

I am so grateful for my healthy upbringing! It wasn't that Mum had us on a diet, it was because she was conscious of healthy eating, and it just grew on us.

I knew there was something important missing in all this healthy eating though, and that was the knowledge of how to put it all together. What we didn't know then but we do know now is that eating 'healthily' isn't necessarily going to give you the body shape of your dreams. A lot of potentially healthy food is often loaded with carbohydrates [carbs] and unhealthy fats, and often the product – fish, for example – is great to start with, but when it's fried and served with fries for dinner, it's lethal!

I actually thought [along with thousands of other teenagers] that the only way to lose weight quickly was to just stop eating. My poor Mum. Can you imagine? What hope did she have trying to convince her teenage daughter [who knew everything – of course] not to do this to her body! But now I realize, with hindsight, that I had so many excellent alternatives.

1987 was a heavy year for this teenage girl. My father suffered terribly from heart problems – he had unstable angina and a 90% closure of his left ventricle. This was caused by heredity, smoking for more than 30 years, and long-term bad eating habits. My Grandma was a single mum of eleven kids during the Depression, as my Grandpa died when my Dad was just ten years old. This meant Grandma had to live on what you could call a tight budget. Carbs and fat came cheap!

It was hard for Dad to change his childhood eating habits. Even though Mum would prepare semi-healthy food, there would always be room for a few slices of bread and butter as well. Dad's weaknesses were chocolate and starchy carbohydrates. And if he had a roast dinner it would be dripping in lots of dripping [fat].

What happened to my Dad shocked us all. It truly transformed our entire family's lifestyle for the better. My father survived major open-heart surgery and is alive and well today, more than 20 years down the track.

Sitting by his bedside taught me something worthwhile: we can change our lives and the quality of them by making certain choices. Mum spent hours, days and weeks, seeking out and modifying all kinds of new recipes and cooking methods.

She turned all the healthiest recipe books upside down, to modify what seemed healthy, to what was actually going to be healthy. Nothing was going to get in the way of reducing my Dad's cholesterol and weight. And, although she isn't a doctor, dietitian or even a personal trainer, she's smart and determined, and she did it!

Mum achieved amazing results by modifying the amount of carbohydrates and eliminating unhealthy fats and an overload of sugar from my Dad's diet. Not only did my father's cholesterol shrink to a very low level, but his body shape changed dramatically, and he had the energy and enthusiasm of a man at least ten years his junior. Dad's doctor, Sydney cardiologist Dr David Baron, was astounded at the short amount of time it took Mum to get Dad's cholesterol and weight down before his urgent heart operation.

Notice how I say Mum did a lot of the work. Dr Baron knew that with Dad's poor eating background he would need my Mum to make the effort. Not everyone is as fortunate as my Dad, to have a 'personal chef' who is so good to him!

It is, however, more than possible for anyone who reads this book to adopt a healthy motivational attitude that will allow them to set and achieve their very own healthy body shaping goals.

My entire family enjoyed the benefits of cutting down on carbohydrates and eliminating unhealthy fats and an overload of sugar. I, for one, was trim and taut and happy to be me. The last thing on my mind was dieting. It just seemed not to be an issue any more. I figured we had this healthy living thing sewn up.

I began modeling at the age of twenty. Even though I always had a steady stream of work [mainly runway], I still lacked confidence. I had a serious self-image problem from all the years of yoyo dieting.

I think it's important at this point to let you know that I never weighed two-hundred-and-something pounds. The sort of weight I am talking about gaining amounts to a couple of dress sizes up and down. That is not to say that if you are more than a few sizes larger than your desired weight that this lifestyle won't work for you – it will.

Although I am now in my 40's, what worked in my 20's still works now, and that is what is so rewarding about the Body & Soul Lifestyle! It is truly worthwhile to wake up every morning and not be consumed about wishing life could be different. I put the effort in and now I am able to reap the reward for all my hard work. Hard work that is fruitless is completely de-motivating. But hard work that produces results is awesome!

> The majority of people in the western world aren't obese – they are just a few sizes bigger that they would like to be.

The Body & Soul Lifestyle has been designed in such a way that it is as effective in dropping the odd pound as it is in dropping 80 pounds or even more.

After beginning work in the 90's with one of Sydney's leading personal training companies, I learned some interesting facts about body shaping. Because I wasn't all that excited by what I saw in the mirror, I set a new goal and I knew I couldn't [and didn't want to] starve myself to do it!

I took out my bathroom scales, my tape measure and my favorite pair of jeans! This would be my new winning combination. Because muscle tissue weighs up to three times more than fat and I knew I was losing fat and gaining muscle, I also knew my scales may appear a little discouraging. That is why my scales and my tape measure and my favorite pair of jeans would be my staple measuring guide. Each week, I would try on my favorite jeans until they fit like a comfy glove. They went from 'breathe-in-and-squeeze-and-forget-it', to 'they're-on-but-don't-ask-me-to-sit-down', to ' Wow!-I-feel-fantastic! Reaching this goal was so incredibly rewarding! I set my goal – and I achieved it without swaying! I lost inches and felt wonderful. It took a complete focus of mind and a determination. I had to make choices to reach my goal.

> If I can lose 5 pounds, I can lose 10
> If I can lose 10 pounds, I can lose 20.
> If I can lose 20 pounds, I can lose anything!

I applied the Body & Soul principles, together with a healthy eating plan where I was having five small meals a day, plus walking. I fully achieved my goal.

I don't care to count the number of years I spent nearly killing myself in aerobic classes in the 80's and 90's, week in, and week out. It wasn't until I slowed down and took part in some steady exercise, at the rate my body worked best, that I saw the fat burning results I wanted.

I continued modeling right up until I was three months pregnant with my twin boys, Bentley and Beau. Knowing that fat cells can be established and stored four times through a woman's life – early childhood, adolescence, pregnancy and menopause – I knew that if I kept my fat intake to a minimum while pregnant, I wouldn't have to work so hard afterwards. I did, however, increase my healthy eating!

I started writing this book back then. I can recall so many times I had to stop writing and run to the bathroom, because I had such awful morning-afternoon-night sickness! I didn't think I'd ever finish writing recipes! The thought of food used to make me so ill.

Thinking back to the early morning starts – sometimes 4.30 am, when I would be standing in my kitchen, barefoot and very pregnant, preparing lunch for some clients
– I have to laugh. It's so rewarding seeing the fantastic results that were achieved. But even with the knowledge I'd already gained, I put on 88 pounds during the pregnancy. By the end of the pregnancy I'd reached 220 pounds and outgrown XXL maternity clothes. It took me until the boys were 18 months old before it was all gone!

Sadly, I found myself a single mom of my twin boys when they were just young toddlers – something that I never dreamt would happen to me. I have so much compassion for people in the same situation. One thing that I have learned first hand is that it's okay to have a new beginning. A wonderful new beginning for me and also for my boys was meeting and marrying the man of my dreams, Jonathan William Wilson. Jonathan is a wonderful man and we love 'doing life' together. Jonathan and his beautiful daughter Rachel [who's now my beautiful daughter!] and Jonathan's wonderful son Joshua [who's now my wonderful son], have brought real joy and a sense of completion to our lives.

I have since given birth to our beautiful daughter, Bella Elena, and I gained the same weight again. I was 30 years old when Bella was born and I thought that the weight would stay on forever. It took a little longer, but eventually I got back in shape.

Then the surprise of my life at the age of 39 I found out I was pregnant again! Another little girl, London Eternity. I didn't quite put on as much weight with this pregnancy, but I did top the scales at 190 pounds. And the hardest part was how much more I wanted to eat while I was nursing. I put on nearly 20 pounds more after London was born. And at the age of 40 I knew I was going to have to work hard to get the weight off and keep it off.

We had just moved from Australia to the USA five months earlier, to start a brand new church [Newport Church in Newport Beach California], so it was an extremely busy season of our lives. We hadn't planned on having another baby, although there was always that niggling feeling that maybe there was one more to come. Maybe there was a little one knocking on Heaven's door to join us down here on earth!

When London Eternity burst onto the scene I can remember realizing that I would have to go through the whole expansion and contraction experience again – and I don't just mean in the labor ward of the hospital. I knew that I would probably gain a huge amount of weight and have to get back in shape once again.

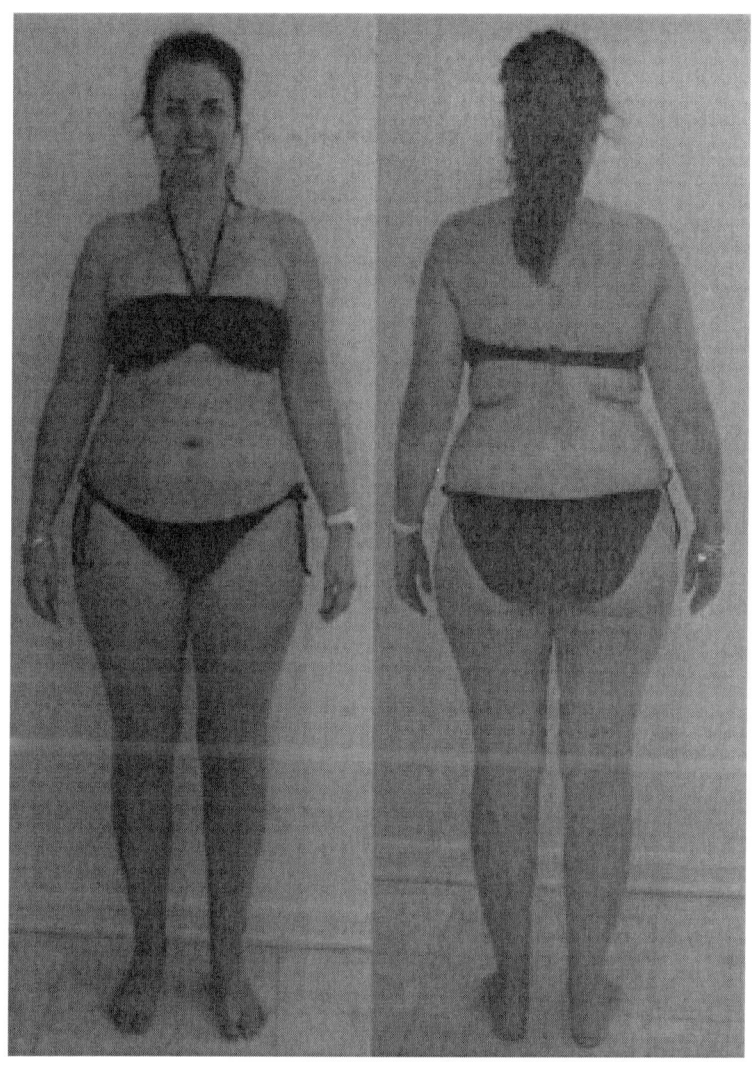

Here I am...
I had already lost 25 pounds.
Just 7 months later, I was back in shape, 75 pounds gone!

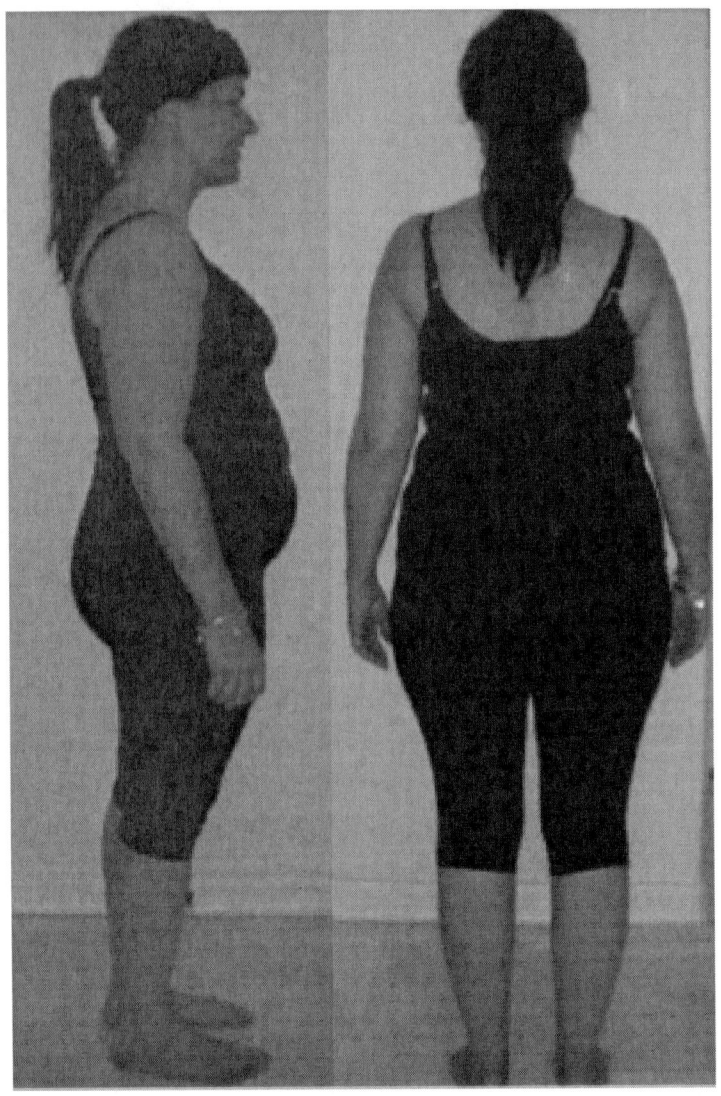

Here I am again …
I had already lost 25 pounds.
Just 7 months later, I was back in shape, 75 pounds gone!

At the age of 40 though, I wasn't sure if I could do it or not. I knew I had the mental focus to at least try, but would my body be able to do it again? That was the question.

I will never forget how difficult it was to walk up and down the stairs, and how painful it was to just turn over in bed at night. Even though I'm tall and can carry a little more weight than someone not as tall, my bone structure is small and the extra weight took its toll on my joints, causing so much daily pain.

When I was younger, being in shape Body & Soul was more about how I looked. Now, in my 40's, being in shape Body & Soul is more about how I feel, even more than how I look. That is something worth putting effort in for.

I've never found that weight just 'falls off'. I haven't found any lying around my house, and when I go for a walk down the street, I haven't seen any falling to the ground! I have always had to 'get rid of it' with purpose and precision. If that's true for you, I'm sure you too will really benefit from the Body & Soul Lifestyle.

I went to a specialized medical weight loss clinic to ask for their assistance. Not because I needed more information [although that is always useful], but because I needed to know that I could do it and having someone in my life to help me through the initial stages was really helpful. After I lost the first 25 pounds, I then interviewed some personal trainers, and found the best in the world! My trainer is so amazing that even after I reached my goal size and weight, I decided to keep her in my life.

Every time I have expanded and contracted in my physical being, I recognize that God has a purpose in every season of my life. I guess my life's story is really my strength. Although I always try to identify with people's pain, I'm not prepared to leave people in their pain. It's great to identify with a problem, but that's not enough to fix it. It's my heart's desire to motivate and encourage you, so you can really enjoy seeing the results – long-term.

The Body & Soul Lifestyle will help you specifically with WHAT to do, WHEN to do it, and HOW it should be done. And, most importantly, you will find out WHY.

Finding the keys to this great lifestyle has been a great learning process for me, and a combination of effort and determination, but it has all paid off. What does a key do? It unlocks something. Throughout the pages of this book you will find many keys that will help you unlock Body & Soul truths, so that you can walk freely through the doors of opportunity provided for you.

After reading and following the Body & Soul Lifestyle, you will also know there is always a point of reference to come back to – a balance – Body & Soul! Even if you're pregnant, sick, or just completely off the rails for a while with your eating, it's always here to come back to.

One thing that is undeniable in my life is that my close relationship with God is the 'secret to my success'. God has given me the ability to change my way of life, and I know you can, too. I know that faith is being sure of what I hoped for, even though I couldn't see the results yet. It's definitely a combination of 'faith' and 'hard work'. We know that faith without work is devoid of power... We must be prepared to work hard, pray for God's help, and believe we will succeed.

Working with people of all different sizes and shapes has made me determined to find out all there is to know about what makes great bodies great. Through study and working closely with a number of body shaping experts, I became aware of a phenomenon. It is not only eating unhealthy fats and an overload of sugar that contributes to weight gain, but eating too many carbohydrates of any description and not enough protein will also rob us of the healthy body shape we desire.

> When the WHY is low the cost is high.
> When the WHY Is high the cost is low.
> Always keep the WHY HIGH.

I also know that increasing cardiovascular activity [walking, cycling, stepper, elliptical, etc] also aids greatly in the fight for a better body shape. The Body & Soul Lifestyle for eating, combined with exercise will give you what you desire. Remember consistency is everything!

I may be in my 40's now, but I lost the weight [75 pounds] after giving birth to my baby girl London Eternity, in half the time. An advantage of being a little more mature is that you realize that you don't want or have time to waste. This time around I wanted to get back in shape faster [without cheating of course], and I have successfully reached my goal. I am asked often how I did it... yes I don't eat unhealthy fats and I don't overload on sugar anymore, and yes I limit the amount of carbohydrates I eat every day and yes I eat a good amount of lean protein and I don't miss any meals or snacks. And yes, I exercise and love the benefits, Body & Soul. But the biggest key to my success is CONSISTENCY. Don't underestimate the power of your daily, moment-by-moment, decisions.

If I can do it, with four kids at home and a super busy life, then trust me, you can do it!

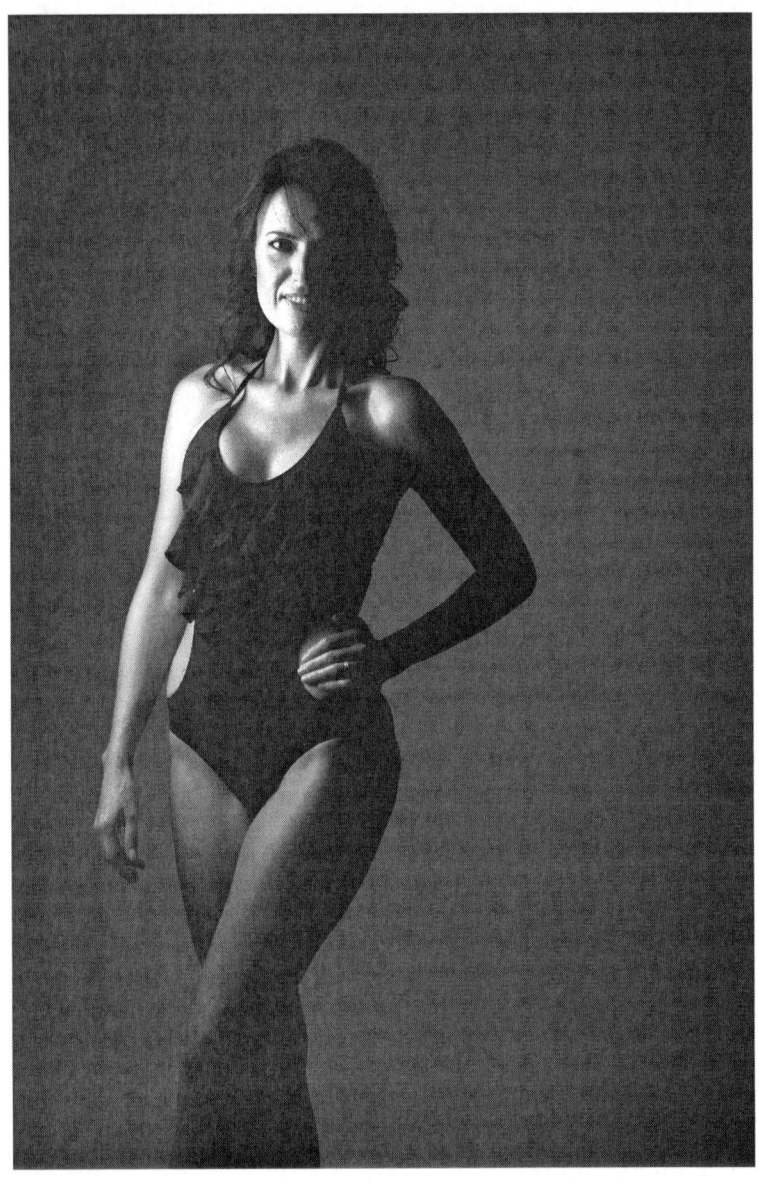

I believe in you…

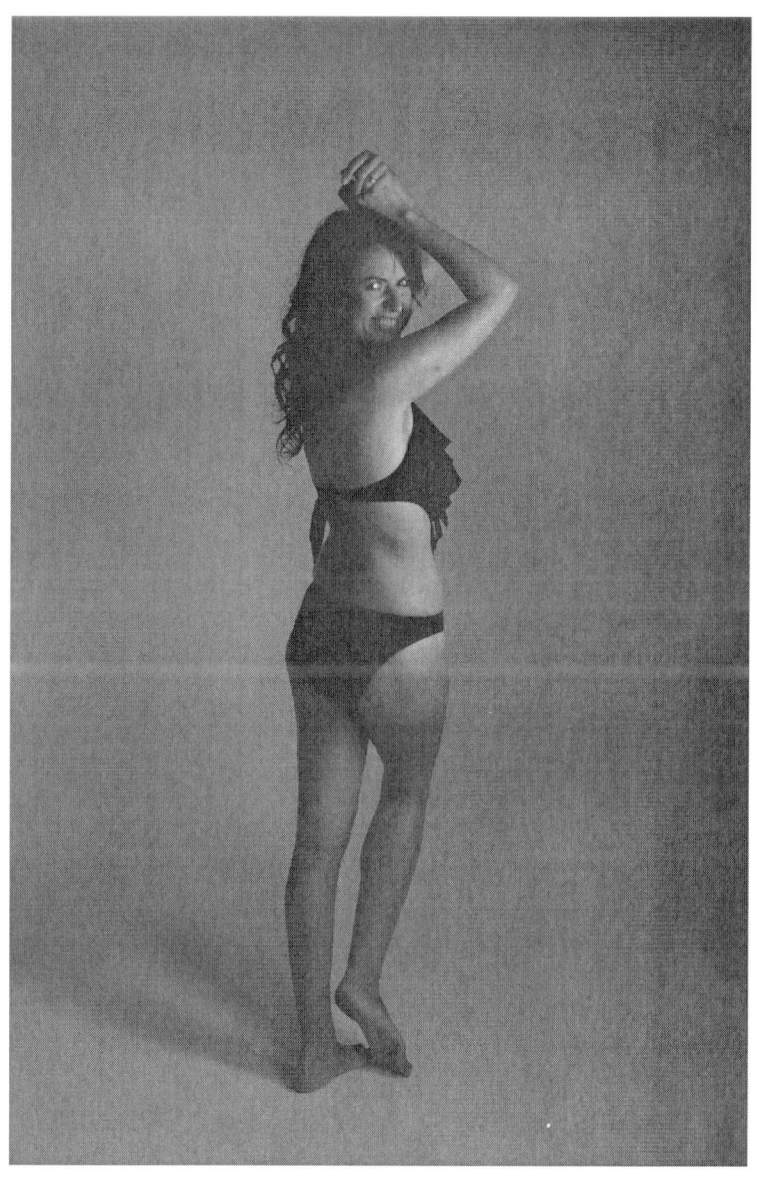

If I can do it... YOU can do it!

Introduction

A short preliminary passage in a larger movement or work.

If someone told you there is a way to get in shape and stay in shape, and it comes down to a simple equation – you'd do it, wouldn't you?

Although I have worked as a personal trainer, it is not the only background to this book. It's more than that. It's trial and error, my experiences and those of other people. After all, who has ever changed by simply knowing something but not applying it to their life?

My experience is that people want to know WHAT to do, WHEN to do it, and exactly HOW it should be done. I wrote Body & Soul for you. Most people are busy and often disheartened by countless failed attempts at dieting. All they really want is to be healthy, look great, and eat well – for good.

> Burn more calories than you eat.
> Do the math –
> It all adds up in your favor – eventually!

My theory is, if you can see the fat, it's too much. As there are enough natural fats in foods, I have designed recipes and methods around utilizing this minimal amount of unseen fat in cooking. Not one recipe has any added butter or cream. The only fat I recommend that you add is a small amount of olive oil or fish oil.

I've created plenty of Body & Soul recipes to tempt any taste-bud, lighten the load off any heart, and to shape any body. What's also unique about this book is its coding system. Each recipe is coded for the best time of day to eat a particular meal. The codes are user friendly, and play a helpful role in the Body & Soul Lifestyle.

As your metabolism works more efficiently earlier in the day, I want to encourage you to eat larger meals earlier in the day and smaller, lighter meals in the evening.

It's not just what you eat [although that is very obviously important], but also the time of day you eat, is vital to a healthier you. This is one of the absolute keys to getting your body into great shape, and is explained in detail throughout the book.

Anyone who's been on any type of diet will be happily surprised at the amount of food I am suggesting should be eaten each day. Often people under-eat, which causes the slowing down of their metabolism, which in turn causes the storage of body fat to increase. This is what the method of 'starving to be slim' can do!

You cannot take off your body
what you keep putting in your mouth.

The whole aim of a personal training service is to provide personal service. The reason this book is different from other books on this subject is that Body & Soul has been produced in the style of a personal training manual, which will enable you to adapt the Body & Soul principles to your lifestyle and make it personal to you.

It's simple once you understand it. The WHAT, WHEN, HOW and WHY of the Body & Soul Lifestyle contained in this book are uncomplicated. Let me ask you a few questions... What have you been eating lately? Do you eat breakfast? Do you know your proteins from your carbohydrates? Do you even care? It is positively vital that you understand your body and what's going into it.

Just as an instruction manual is very handy and necessary to repair a television or video, we could have done well with a Body & Soul instruction manual at birth. It's simple reality that we just don't know enough about our bodies, so we therefore can't expect the best from them. Body & Soul can become your body shaping training manual. I have found that the best manual for life however, is God's Word - the Bible as it feeds, directs and inspires us spirit, soul and body.

> Without involvement, there's no commitment.
> Mark it down, asterisk it, circle it, underline it.
> No involvement, no commitment!
> Stephen R. Covey

You may be familiar with the Healthy Food Pyramid, or the Five Food Groups that were taught at school. What you need to do now is keep them as a reference point, but remember: the more specificity with which you utilize each food group, the better your results will be. We will explore the wonderful world of the body shaping food groups. I don't believe square pegs should have to be squeezed into round holes, so you will learn how to adapt these Body & Soul principles into YOUR BODY and YOUR LIFE.

Once we understand that we can't just pray or wish our problems away and that we need to also take action, it puts us in a better frame of mind to succeed.

The Body & Soul Lifestyle is written in three easy stages for you to follow:

The Body & Soul Lifestyle

STAGE 1: LIFESTYLE PRINCIPLES:
Easy to adapt lifestyle principles
Body & Soul

STAGE 2: FOOD:
What you should eat and when, including great Body & Soul Recipes

STAGE 3: EXERCISE:
Body shaping exercise to give you the body of your dreams

Remember, I believe in you! You can do this!

I once read a Bible verse – 3 John 1:2, personally paraphrased that I would love to share with you...

"Beloved one, I pray to God and wish on account of each and every bit of your life, regarding all things, that

you, loved one, have a successful life and journey, and that your body be free from injury and disease, that you are sound and well, in direct proportion to having your mind, will and emotions prospered and flourishing."

That is my prayer for you – that you would know that God is with you, Body & Soul, and that with every prayer you pray and every effort you put in, He will be there to partner with you to help you achieve your goals. I know because I couldn't have done what I have done without Him!

Life is full of choices.

5 Basic Body & Soul Keys to Remember

1. If you eat often, you will help your body burn fat.

2. By increasing your lean protein intake, you will maintain muscle, and that will help burn fat.

3. By cutting down on starchy and sugary carbohydrates, you will store less fat.

4. Do steady, focused exercise, and you will burn fat and shape up.

5. Walk and pray – do both and you will prosper, Body & Soul.

I've done the lot – and now it's your turn!

Welcome to the freedom that the Body & Soul Lifestyle brings!

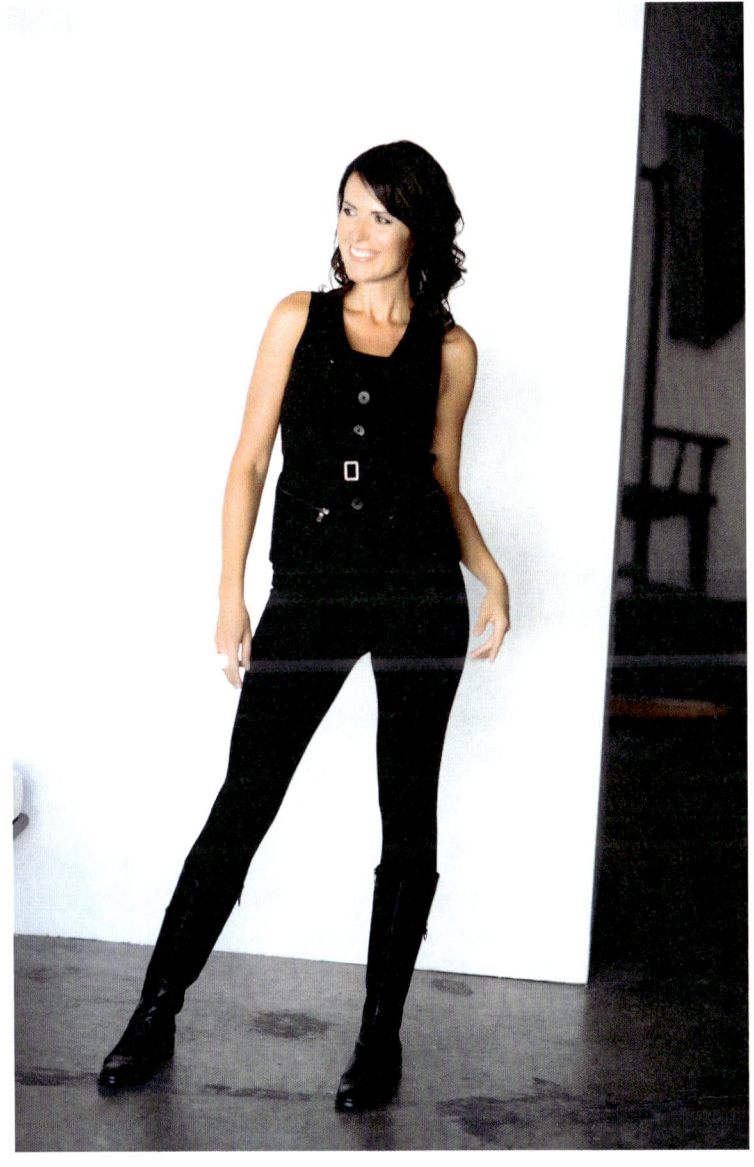

Choose life.

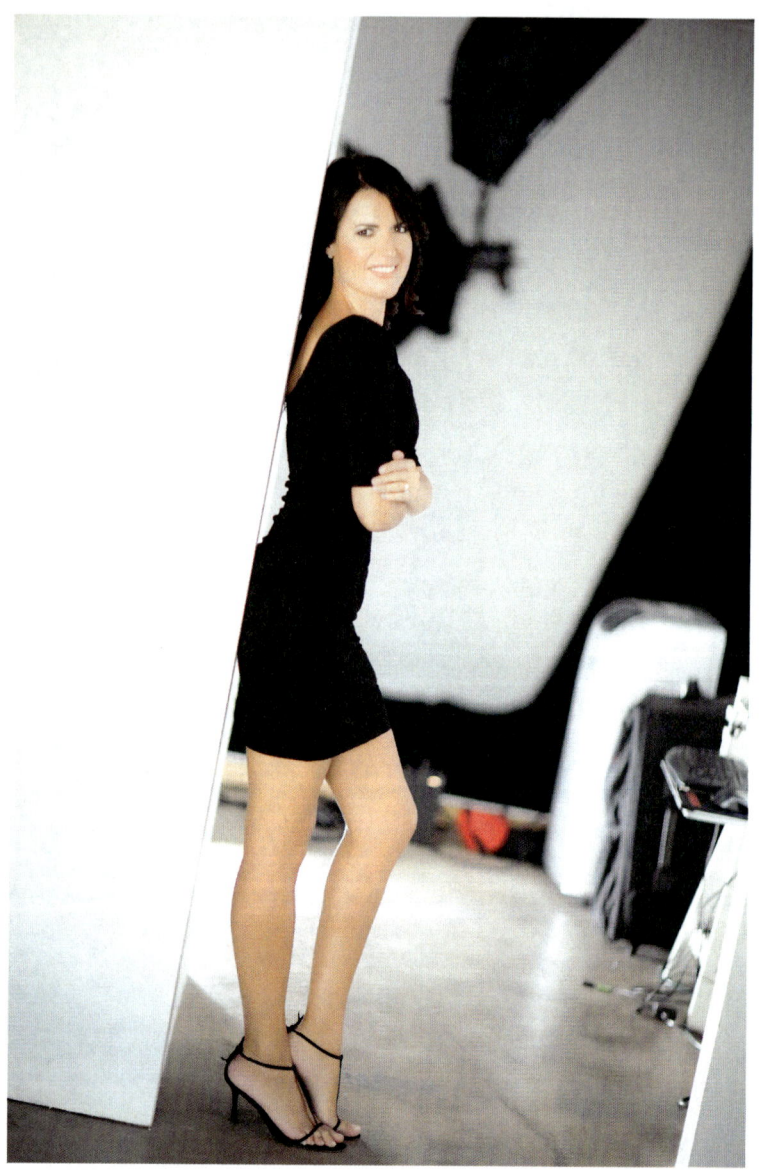

Principles … life's essential ingredients.

Stage

Lifestyle Principles

Lifestyle Principles

★ **Body, Soul and Spirit**

★ **True Confessions**

★ **Freedom Forever!**

★ **Great Expectations**

★ **Establish Your Enemies**

★ **Body Types and Metabolism**

★ **Motivate Me!**

★ **Commitment**

★ **Consistency**

Chapter

1

Body, Soul and Spirit

The three complete components of a person.

> Beloved, I pray that you may prosper in all things and be in health, just as your soul prospers.
> 3 John 1:2

There is a perfect harmony and balance that we can find for our lives when our body, soul and spirit are in sync, healthy and prospering. The Bible tells us in Genesis 1 that we are created in the image and likeness of God, body, soul and spirit. That is God's original blueprint for our lives: three parts working together, creating a magnificent and beautiful synergy. Without all three parts working together we will never be able to realize our full potential in life.

Although it is possible to have a highly developed spiritual life and connection with God, it doesn't mean we will automatically be able to enjoy the fullness and potential of it, especially if we have not taken care of our physical bodies. We will never be able to fulfill our destiny, enjoy our families, longevity and the rewards of our work, if our lives are cut short or impaired by poor health as a result of neglect of our body.

It is also possible to have a healthy body but never reach our full potential because the spiritual dimension of our life has been ignored. The results of ignoring or neglecting our spirit will be a disconnection from God and a *'dis-ease'* in our soul.

It has been widely acknowledged for a long time that a *dis-ease* in our soul is strongly connected to manifestation of physical disease. This is of course not surprising as all three parts of our being, body, soul and spirit, are so closely connected.

We can also have all the ingredients at our disposal to live a healthy spiritual and physical life, but fail to make the right choices and decisions that enable us to realize our potential.

If our body is the temple of the Holy Spirit then our soul is definitely the steering wheel or rudder of our lives. It is the seat of our mind, our will and our emotions, the place where we reason and decide what course of action we will take and stick to. It is the incubator for 'reason' and 'decision making' in our life!

So our soul is the key to directing our minds, our

emotions and our will towards God as our source of strength, life and inspiration, and to making the decisions to do what it takes to live a healthy life – Body, Soul and Spirit

> For as a person thinks in their heart,
> so they will be.
> Proverbs 23:7

Real change works from the inside out!

What we think is what we will become!

What we feed is what will grow!

If physical food feeds our body, then we need to realize there is soul food that can feed our soul and spiritual food that can feed our spirit. We also need to realize that the 'junk in, junk out' principle applies to every area of our lives: body, soul and spirit!

If we want to get the best out of our life, we need to be putting the best in! Therefore, by connecting with God's Spirit, our spirit comes to life and we change from the inside out. When we read God's Word - the Bible, we are fed spiritually and our faith grows and feeds our soul. If we don't feed our spirit on a healthy spiritual 'diet' our faith won't grow, and where there is an absence of faith, fear which is the opposite of faith, is free to grow.

If our soul is choked by fear it will be much harder for us to get into shape physically. Fear that you can't do it, fear that you have no self-control, fear that you will fail, fear that others will judge you, fear that you'll never be able to change your life the way you want to.

The truth is, what we believe and how we think

completely affects how our body responds.

> Fear is an acid which is pumped
> into one's atmosphere.
> It causes mental, moral, and spiritual asphyxiation,
> and sometimes death –
> death of energy and all growth.
> - Horace Fletcher

Faith, however, speaks a different language.

- Faith says, "I can do all things through Christ who gives me strength…"
- Faith says, "all things are possible to those who believe…"
- Faith says, "this moment is the most important moment of my life because my future will not be defined by what happened yesterday but by what I decide today…"

We begin to act as we think. That is why when we align our thinking with God's thinking and fill our minds with what God's Word - the Bible - says, we can grow stronger and healthier, spirit, soul and body every day. When we feed our body, soul and spirit with the right things and our thinking is healthy, we will also be able to deal with life's stresses and pressures without being taken out or getting off course.

Our reactions and responses will begin to change and fall in line with our new Body & Soul Lifestyle. Instead of reaching for comfort food when a crisis hits, or stopping eating altogether, we will start making the right choices and responses in those challenging seasons.

A well-nourished spirit and soul will have a dramatic

effect on our health. A healthy spirit clearly leads to a healthy soul, which helps us work on a healthy body.

Every one of us is uniquely different in body, in soul and in spirit. Just as there is no-one else with your identical finger prints - not even an identical twin - the same applies to your soul and your spirit.

You are created in the image and likeness of God. And He is a uniquely creative God who thought to make you absolutely different and unique to anyone else in the world. In fact, He decided to bring you to earth because He didn't have one of YOU and He decided that you would bring color and flavor to the world, and this world wouldn't be the same without YOU. You have been created for a purpose bigger than you may realize, and that is why it is so important to be healthy and strong in body, in soul and in spirit.

I've learned in life that real change starts on the inside of us and works its way out. God's work of changing us begins in our spirit. Our spirit is that unseen internal part of us that makes us truly alive and distinguishes between right and wrong. When God speaks to us, He speaks to our spirit. It is our spirit that is the starting point of God's relationship with us, and where we hear the sound of His voice.

If we don't have a personal relationship with God through the Lord Jesus Christ, then we won't understand the life and power of our spirit. Our spirit allows us to believe before we see. Our spirit allows us to know truth and walk in relationship with God. This means that we can know a genuine and powerful partnership that will fuel our efforts. I personally would not have been able to do what I have done without being able to partner with God.

> The Life of Freedom...
> Christ has set us free to live a free life.
> So take your stand!
> Never again let anyone
> put a harness of slavery on you.
> Galatians 5:1-3 in The Message

Perhaps you recognize that you don't have a personal relationship with God through having asked the Lord Jesus Christ to live in your heart. If you want to trade in 'religion' for a genuine relationship, you can make that change today.

Knowing God is not about joining a religion, following a set of rules, or even about being a "good person". Knowing Him is about having your own personal relationship with the Creator of the universe, discovering just how much He truly loves you, and embarking on the journey of loving Him back.

In uncertain times and as our own personal trials persist – God is with us. He has promised to never leave us or forsake us, to walk with us through the valleys of life, and to rejoice with us during times of celebration.

The fact is, God loves us.

He loves you.

The Bible says that He loves you so much that He sent His Son, Jesus Christ, to die for you, and stand in the gap for all of our sins. The Bible also says that no matter what our past has been like or what bad decisions we have made, we are forgiven when we give our lives to Christ. We can have a fresh start on life and a hope for the future!

Jesus is our connection to God and to His grace. It is through a personal relationship with Him that we are saved. Not by our own striving, not by anything we have done [or not done] – it's all about having a real relationship with Him. A relationship is what He wants from us, and the Bible says that when we draw near to Him, He draws near to us. And that's good news!

My prayer for you is that you may you know Him. May you know His love – and may you be overwhelmed as you watch Him do things with your life that will far exceed anything you could ask, hope or dream!

If you have never had a relationship with Jesus, or perhaps you once did, but you're now away from Him, right now I want to encourage you to pray this prayer:

> *Dear Jesus,*
> *Right now, I want to make the decision to stop living my life my own way, and begin living it Your way.*
> *I ask that You would forgive me for all my sins, give me a brand new start today and hope for my future.*
> *I want to be a Christian, a follower of Jesus Christ, for the rest of my life.*
> *Amen!*

If you have just prayed this prayer for the first time, or have rededicated your life to Christ, congratulations! I would love to hear from you! Please take a moment to email me at dianne@diannewilson.com, so I can help you take steps on this new journey of really knowing God, body, soul and spirit.

Chapter

2

True Confessions

An open profession of faith that works.

The way we think is absolutely crucial to our success in life. That is why I am including this chapter, to help you start your brand new Body & Soul Lifestyle from a position of strength. Even if you have tried and failed or tried, succeeded and then failed in the past, today is a new day. It's a blank canvas for you to decide who you want to be, how you want to feel and look, and what you want your future to be like.

Positive confession is amazing for our soul and our body, as we reaffirm truth and agree with what our Creator says about us. This has been such a crucial part of my own personal success, especially when difficult seasons arise. It isn't enough for us to think positive thoughts, we need to confess positive confessions from the Word of God. When doubt fills our hearts, it is often difficult to embark on a new path. Doubt is a well-worth trench that wants to pull us backwards in life. We need to jump onto a new path of faith that says we can do this!

Following are 10 True Confessions found in the Word of God – the Bible. Read and believe!

10 True Confessions

1. **I am Created in the image and likeness of God**
   "So God created man in His own image, in the image and likeness of God He created him; male and female He created them."
   [Genesis 1:27]

2. **I am fearfully and wonderfully made**
   "For you created my inmost being; you knit me together in my mother's womb. I praise you because I am fearfully and wonderfully made; your works are wonderful, I know that full well.
   My frame was not hidden from you when I was made in the secret place. When I was woven together in the depths of the earth…"
   [Psalm 139:13-15]

3. **I am free**
   "So if the Son liberates you [makes you free men], then you are really and unquestionably free."

[John 8:36]

4. **I am loved**
"Dear friends, since God so loved us, we also ought to love one another."
[1 John 4:11]

5. **I am accepted**
"Accept one another, then, just as Christ accepted you, in order to bring praise to God."
[Romans 15:7]

6. **I am valuable**
"For God so loved the world that he gave his one and only Son, that whoever believes in him shall not perish but have eternal life."
[John 3:16]

7. **I am blessed**
"And my God will liberally supply [fill to the full] your every need according to His riches in glory in Christ Jesus."
[Philippians 4:19]

8. **I am intelligent**
"For who has known or understood the mind [the counsels and purposes] of the Lord so as to guide and instruct Him and give Him knowledge? But we have the mind of Christ [the Messiah] and do hold the thoughts [feelings and purposes] of His heart."
[1 Corinthians 2:16]

9. **I have hope**
   "For I know the thoughts and plans that I have for you, says the Lord, thoughts and plans for welfare and peace and not for evil, to give you hope in your final outcome."
   [Jeremiah 1:29]

10. **I am strong**
    "I have strength for all things in Christ Who empowers me [I am ready for anything and equal to anything through Him Who infuses inner strength into me; I am self-sufficient in Christ's sufficiency]."
    [Philippians 4:13]

Amen!

Chapter

3

Freedom Forever!

The power to determine action without restraint.

Here's a thought that most people can relate to: I do what I know I shouldn't do and I don't do what I know I should do.

It's a very common human dilemma.

We know what we shouldn't do. We shouldn't:

- binge eat
- not eat
- eat and throw up or take laxatives
- eat too much junk
- eat unhealthy fats
- sit around doing nothing
- tell ourselves we're fat, ugly and useless!

Many of us also know what it is that we should do. We should:

- eat right
- exercise
- believe we can do it!

> What I don't understand about myself is that
> I decide one way, but then act another,
> doing things I absolutely despise...
> I realize that I don't have what it takes.
> I can will it, but I can't do it.
> I decide to do good, but I don't really do it;
> I decide not to do bad, but then I do it anyway.
> My decisions, such as they are, don't result in actions.
> Romans 7 in The Message

So how do we get free forever?!

I want you to say the following statement out loud, to yourself: 'I'm not perfect, and I don't have to be either!'

In the game called LIFE, there are rules we have to play by. For every action or game play in life, there is either a positive or a negative reaction or consequence. If we don't play according to the rules, we suffer the consequences. It's our choice.

Life is full of good and bad choices, but it's also full of good and bad consequences. It's an inescapable fact. If you overeat or under-eat, on a regular basis, you'll not only bear the fruit of that behavior by becoming overweight or underweight, but you will also be guilt-ridden and bound in your conscience, because you've crossed the line that you were never meant to cross. Life is meant to be lived and enjoyed. It's also meant to be fruitful. If your life is anything but enjoyable and fruitful, perhaps it's time to take stock and look at what is holding you back.

My mission in life is to see you set free so that you can live your life the way you were created to live: healthy in body, soul and spirit.

We were all born into this world full of potential. The sense of that potential is so evident in young children that it can sometimes come as a shock. I remember once after saying to my daughter Bella when she was just four years old, "You're beautiful", and she said back to me, "Yes Mummy".

I remember it surprising me for a moment. I then thought about it. There is absolutely no reason on earth why Bella wouldn't believe she is beautiful. She was four years old and all she's been told is that she is beautiful. No-one has put her down; she hasn't put herself down. Life hasn't knocked the 'stuffing' out of her.

We've all felt at times that we have been knocked over, but we don't need to be knocked out. Picture one of those silly clowns that, no matter how many times you hit it, bounces back to the upright position. If it's easy enough for a plastic clown, it should be easy enough for us. Just don't let your feet ever leave the ground!

To some people, being a few pounds overweight is enough to put them in a spin. Others can be 50 pounds overweight and be completely oblivious to how dangerous it is to their health. It's all relative. I don't like being a few pounds overweight, let alone being 50 or more pounds overweight. I had to really watch my thoughts when I put on a lot of weight, especially with my last pregnancy. I had to be careful not to take on the mindset of ' obesity', although my weight was right up there! All this would do would be to keep me trapped further and longer.

Talk about a treadmill! Some people are on a treadmill 24 hours a day, 7 days a week, 365 days a year. But it's the, *'I need to do something about my body but can't seem to get motivated variety!'* That's a treadmill I want to help you get off!

> Body & Soul
> is not about perfection.
> It's about freedom.

Something that I have learned is that putting a name to something gives it an identity. When I was a teenager, my eating was rather disorderly, or not in order. But I didn't consider myself to have an eating disorder. There is a difference between disorderly eating and an eating disorder. The difference is in the crossing of the line. I had mild anorexia, but didn't recognize it. To me, it's what Karen Carpenter died of, and that wasn't going to happen to me!

There is a point at which a line is crossed, and that line is either into the 'over' [obesity/binge eating] category, or into the ' under' [anorexia/bulimia] category. I basically played near the 'under' line as a teenager, but I never crossed over to the point of no return. There is a big difference, and that's why people find it difficult and sometimes impossible to cross back over that line.

For example, on a scale of 1 to 10, with 1 being mild and 10 being severe, you may have an issue relating to the way you look and feel. Even a score of 1 or 2 means that you are not completely free. A score of 1 or 2 is enough to stop most people from fulfilling their potential in life.

After the birth of Bella and then after the birth of London, I was up very close to the 'over' line. It would have been easy to cross over and stay overweight forever. I had to make choice after choice to go down, slowly and surely. It's when people cross over the line that the term eating disorder really applies.

Eating disorders in their various forms are serious and dangerous. At any Body & Soul seminar there are always people who are overweight and also people who are underweight.   I'm very aware of the fact that people struggle at both ends of the spectrum.

I'm also very aware that not every woman or man who is overweight eats more than someone who has a 'typical' body shape. Everyone's metabolism is different and it's really important for us not to judge why someone is larger or smaller than we are.

It's my heart's desire to see people set free in all areas of eating, be it over or under. There is a great need to address this issue before we get into the practical side of the Body & Soul Lifestyle. I call it my mission from the inside out. Sadly, many professionals in the body shaping industry spend most of their time working from the outside to the inside.

'Lose weight, feel great!'
'Lose weight, meet a mate!'
'Lose weight, eat some cake!'
'Lose weight, succeed in life!'

An eating disorder, whether mild or severe, starts somewhere. It is not a physical condition, or even merely an emotional or mental condition. An eating disorder, I believe, starts from a condition of the heart.

All little girls dream of being princesses. I dreamed about being a princess, although the reality of being a princess was definitely far, far away. I grew up in a very loving home with a very loving family. For any of you who have sisters, you may be able to relate to the normal sibling rivalry I grew up with. Unfortunately though, because my sister was [and still is] a stunning green-eyed blonde, and I am a dark-eyed brunette, the princess theme didn't quite fit my mold.

So, during childhood games, I was relegated to play the part of the prince, or the slave, or even worse, the wicked witch. This was mainly due to the fact that I was the youngest, but back then all I could imagine it was to do with was the color of my hair and eyes – the way I looked.

In the 70's in Australia, the ethnic minority of immigrants weren't treated with a great deal of respect. I know because I was often mistaken for one. I was called 'wog' and other unkind names, which are now very politically incorrect!

At the same time, my parents told me I was beautiful. So rather than becoming confused, wondering who was right and who was wrong, I believed the voice of negativity which told me I was different, which made me feel ugly and unacceptable. I was too young to know any different.

It's laughable now, especially when I look back on many years of career success as a model. I was unusual, I guess – not a classic blonde and blue-eyed Aussie chick. When the dark exotic look came in, and the European influence became more a way of life here, I was booked for a lot of work on the best catwalks the country had to offer. Even though I was receiving a great deal of work as a model, I still struggled with my self-worth.

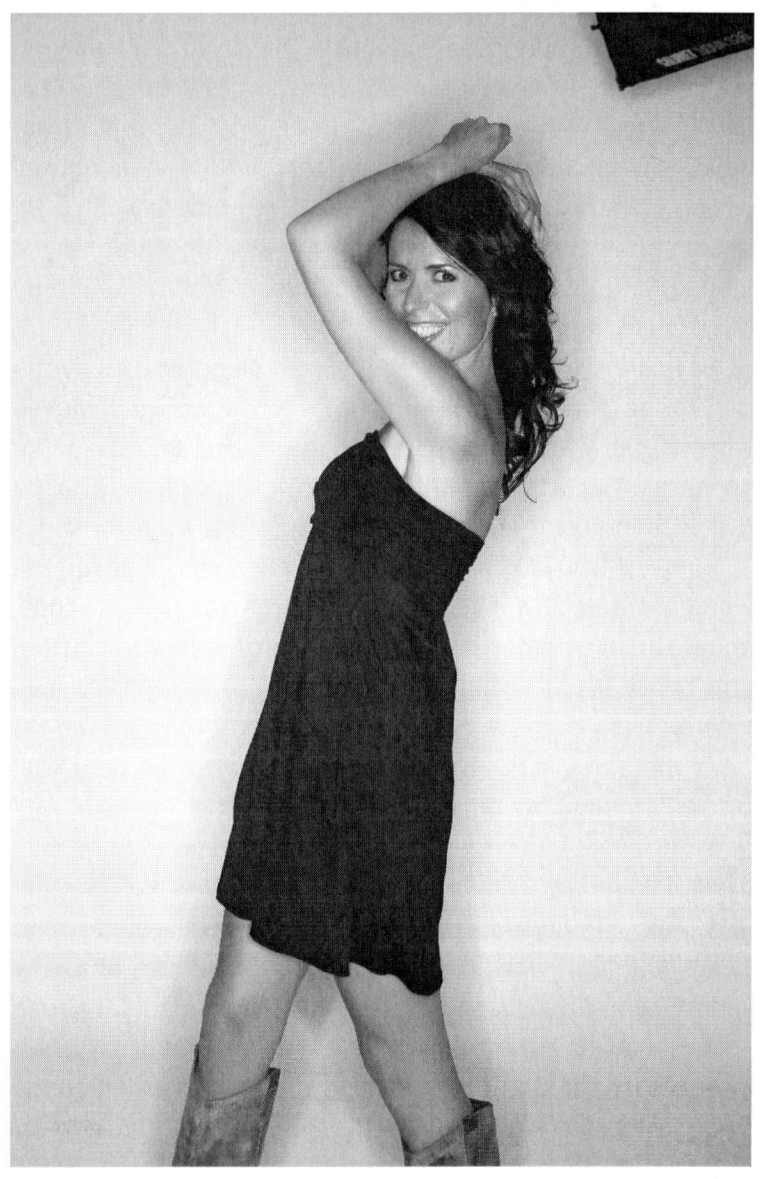

I love being free.

It wasn't really tied up in my looks, or how much money I was paid. It was deeper than that. I needed someone to show me the way to freedom. Personally speaking, everything changed for me at the point when I chose to believe God's Word - the Bible and what it has to say about me, and my life. We can hear truth and walk away and nothing changes. We need to listen to truth and apply what it says, so we can become all that we are on the planet to be. The truth within these pages might just change your life.

The fact that I am a living testimony really helps my endeavor to help you! I have walked this walk and want to show you how beneficial and life changing it can be. My test in life has become my testimony. I love being free!

You may have had an issue with body image, overeating, under-eating, dieting or all of the above. Let's see if we can't smash the chains of entrapment and bring some freedom into your life. It's about time! The first step to take is a 'reality check' on the things that could hold you back.

Some of the things that you may need to deal with are:

- Issues relating to obesity [being more than 20% above the ideal body weight for your age and height].
- Various forms of eating disorders [anorexia, bulimia or binge eating]

Understanding what these things are and working towards removing them and their effects from your life is a top priority. It's important to launch into the Body & Soul lifestyle from a position of strength, that is, having a healthy opinion of yourself. Even if you would like to improve certain aspects of your body shape, it's important to have a healthy body image to begin with.

Body image is basically:

- How you see or picture yourself.
- How you feel that other people perceive you.
- What you see in the mirror and believe.
- How you feel about your physical appearance.

The media has a huge part to play in the negative perceptions of our body image. We are constantly bombarded with 'perfection', and are encouraged to strive for the same. We in the Western world place a high value upon appearance. If you are attractive, you must be worth more. It's just not the truth.

As parents, we need to be very careful about how we conduct ourselves in front of our children, including small children. If we are constantly dieting, or putting ourselves down, what are we saying to our children? Please be mindful and careful.

The world of dieting can be quite overwhelming. Take your mind away from the concept of dieting, and engage it in a complete change of lifestyle. That's what the Body & Soul Lifestyle is all about.

One thing that I have found with people who have suffered from eating disorders is that although they want to be better, they are terribly afraid of getting fat. I can understand that thought process. I honestly can. Most of the people I have met who have suffered from an eating disorder have said the same thing: that the doctors have tried to get them to gain any weight, and thus put them on high fat, high carbohydrate diets.

I believe that there is another solution that will not compromise the health of the individual – body and soul.

The Body & Soul Lifestyle is designed to give people lean muscle gain and fat loss, and for them to have loads of energy. The under-eaters that I have helped with the

Body & Soul Lifestyle have really enjoyed it because it means that they can eat and put on weight, but not put on fat – which is what they are afraid of, and why they have the eating disorder in the first place.

I am not a doctor and I respect those who are. I just don't necessarily agree that the methods of old which are sometimes used currently are going to be of benefit to those who struggle not within their bodies, but with how they see themselves. They don't want to get fat, so I don't believe making them eat lots of fat is going to help them with the way they see themselves! In my opinion, all this does is hinder people from getting free.

Most of us crave chocolate more than we crave freedom! We go for the quick fix. Instant gratification. Short-term gain [the taste of chocolate] and long-term pain [a life of out-of-control eating]. Why? Because as human beings we do what we know we shouldn't do and we don't do what we know we should do. We know what is good and what is bad, but we need to get free. True freedom is about being comfortable in your own skin. Whatever is holding you back needs to be rectified. We need to understand that we need help from a higher source!

> ... I've tried everything and nothing helps.
> I'm at the end of my rope.
> Is there no one who can do anything for me?
> Isn't that the real question?
> The answer, thank God, is that Jesus Christ can and does. He acted to set things right in this life of contradictions..."
> Romans 7 in The Message

Hey! Smile at the future and believe that you can achieve your dreams!

7 Keys to a Healthy Self-Esteem

1. Find something you like about yourself- grow in awareness of your positive attributes.

2. When you buy fashion magazines, decide not to measure yourself against the size 0 models.

3. Eat healthily – follow the Body & Soul Lifestyle.

4. Exercise regularly – you won't know how fantastic you feel until you get out and do it!

5. Replace bad habits with good habits, for life!

6. Be honest with yourself, and refuse to put yourself down. If you can't say something nice about yourself, don't say anything at all.

7. Be grateful for how you were made. Recognize that a bulge to you may be a curve to someone else. Curves are beautiful, so don't despise them.

Chapter

4

Great Expectations

Looking forward to something with enormous anticipation.

You will want to know what you should expect if you follow the Body & Soul Lifestyle. You will lose body fat, retain muscle tissue, lower cholesterol, have increased energy, and you will sleep soundly.

Firstly, if you follow what I've outlined, even if you cannot manage to take part in any exercise, you will lose body fat. Basically, what doesn't go in your mouth – fat – has to come off your body. And what's left underneath the fat is your body's muscle tissue, which gives you your shape – so you don't want to lose it!

Because muscle outweighs fat by three times, it's important not to concern yourself to the point of obsession when weighing in.

> You will eat better, sleep better, work better, feel better and look better.
> And... everyone [who matters] will notice!

A great thing to do is to grab your favorite jeans or piece of clothing that you wish you could fit into, and try it on once a week.

Also, if you can go to the gym and have a body fat test done, you will be surprised at the amount of fat lost after following the Body & Soul Lifestyle for a few weeks. You may not see dramatic results in weight or size loss before then, because you won't be losing water or muscle tissue, which is the bulk of the weight lost on most typical diets.

The reality is that stubborn fat is always the last to leave your body. You will be laying down healthy foundation stones by sticking to the Body & Soul Lifestyle. It's a worthwhile lifestyle investment.

This means that if you lose your way later on, you can always find help again with this lifestyle, and it should only take you about one third of the time to regain your great body shape.

Don't expect the same results you've had with other diets. You may even feel like giving up after a week, but once you've pushed through, around the 21-day mark, you will be firing on all cylinders! It will become a part of you and your lifestyle.

What is so wonderful about the Body & Soul Lifestyle is that you begin to gain freedom from the very first week, if you do exactly what you are supposed to. That means you get to walk out this Lifestyle, whether it is for 6 weeks or 6 months in freedom, rather than hoping that freedom will come once you reach a certain size. Freedom comes when you say you will do something and actually do it! And that will happen the first week if you stay focused!

The body's metabolism is truly remarkable. I liken it to knowing when you need to go to the bathroom. Once your body is in tune with proper eating, it lets you know – loud and clear – when it wants to eat. For the first week or so, you will probably have to keep checking what to eat and when to eat it. After that, your body will let you know what it needs and when.

This lifestyle is part of an education process. I'm educating your mind; it's up to you to educate your body. This is the only way you'll change your body's metabolism into super-turbo mode!

At around the three-week mark, you will start to see a difference, and you will certainly feel different:

"I am sleeping so soundly now."

"I have lots of energy throughout the day."

These comments are from normal, everyday people – not even necessarily those who are able to go to the gym each day to exercise. It's simply due to proper eating.

If you cannot exercise [I know what it's like to have small kids, and how restrictive that can be], this lifestyle will work for you. However, by adding some focused exercise, such as walking for 45 to 60 minutes a day, three to five times a week, you will lose even more body fat. If you are really keen, try to get to a gym where there are proper weights and machines to start sculpting your body.

Everyone wants to know what makes great bodies great. I'm sure you've seen an amazing physique and wondered how the person attained it. I know I have. Yes, genetics have a lot to do with it, but lifestyle is an even greater contributor! We can all improve, and that's what we need to know.

7 Keys to a Improving Your Body Shape

1.   Eliminate unhealthy fats and sugar-rich foods.

2.   Limit the amount of carbohydrates [especially at night] you eat each day.

3.   Increase your intake of lean protein.

4.   Don't miss meals or snacks, every 2 hours.

5.   Drink 5 small bottles of water each day.

6.   Do steady cardio exercise, such as walking, 4-5 days a week.

7.   Lift weights two to three times a week.

This is an optimum plan for an optimum body.

Experiencing amazing results – Body & Soul will help you stay motivated until you reach your goal.

At about the six to eight week mark, even without too much exercise, you will notice a real difference in your body's shape. This will motivate and catapult you into the next phase. I try to only set goals that are around the six to eight week mark – something achievable.

If you know the truth of what to expect at the outset, then the Body & Soul Lifestyle will not only assist your motivation, but you will not stop because you will see the results you want and in the shortest possible time [without cheating of course!]

Imagine setting a body shaping goal and actually achieving it! It does wonders for your self-esteem, not to mention your body shape.

Be realistic in your goal setting, and remember the old saying, "Slow and steady wins the race". It will work for you. Don't be in a big hurry to lose weight too quickly, or else [as usual] it won't stay off.

Sit back and dream about the type of body shape you want and the size you want to be, and then start planning for it.

> Begin with the end in mind.
> Stephen R. Covey

Chapter

5

Establish Your Enemies

A hostile power or harmful force.

Sometimes we are our own worst enemy.

We aren't born that way nor do we mean to be that way, but it can often come about because of our past experiences, what someone may have told us, and then without realizing, we develop inner enemies.

Take confused decision making as an example, where we know we want something but we don't know what that something is, and we are easily confused when presented with options to change.

When we allow confused decision making to rule our life we won't go ahead and commit to anything because we can't recognize clear solutions right in front of our eyes.

Part of the price of achieving our goals is to move outside of our comfort zone and to do some new things that we may not have done before. The reward is that this helps us to grow as a person. It takes us to new heights, while also enabling us to experience adventure and fun.

We need to be willing to meet our enemies face to face and then be courageous enough to kiss them good-bye! This is a war against Body & Soul. We need to know our enemies so that we are ready for combat:

5 Body Shaping Enemies

1.   Too many carbohydrates and not enough lean protein.

2.   Unhealthy fats and an overload of sugar

3.   Dehydration.

4.   Over-exercise or under-exercise.

5.   Not believing in yourself!

These 5 Body Shaping Enemies are a combination that can cause damage. Discontinuing one without the others simply will not help you achieve the body shape of your dreams. These enemies need elimination!

Never befriend these enemies. Hey, I repeat, *never befriend these enemies*. Sugar is addictive, chocolate is addictive and they are enemies that will beckon you to eat them every single day and they will lead you to believe that you can't live without them. See them for what they are – enemies – and eliminate!

The myth surrounding carbohydrates – 'energy foods' – is that you need huge amounts of them to function each day. The only problem with this is that unless you are training like an ironman or elite athlete, you shouldn't be eating breakfast cereal like one! Unless you are extremely active – and 90% of us are not – then energy foods, including bananas, will be stored in your body. This unused glut of energy foods is stored in the form of fat.

Nine times out of ten, if you are feeling lethargic and needing what you think is an energy boost, your body is dehydrated and simply needs a water refueling, and could probably do with a brisk walk around the block!

Firstly, you need to assess your body type [see Body Types and Metabolism, Chapter 6], and only take in food that you need to function healthily, to give you enough fiber and energy to fight the fight against fat, and nothing more.

You may well be watching your unhealthy fats intake and being careful not to overload on sugars, but you also need to be very careful about the amount of carbohydrates you consume every day, and try to minimize them at night.

This will make a big difference in anything you may have tried before.

When it comes to the subject of exercise, it's important to realize that you can be doing the wrong kind of exercise and that will inhibit your body shaping results.

For instance, make sure that when you do cardio exercise, you take it steady and don't get too breathless. Now this doesn't mean that you shouldn't work up a sweat, but it does mean that you should be working at a pace you can sustain, and not have to give up because you used all your energy in the first ten minutes.

One of the greatest body shaping tools I own is a heart rate monitor. It helps me know when I am in fat burning range, and how many calories I burn every time I do cardio or weights. It also helps me stay safe when exercising, so that I don't go overboard.

> It's when things seem worst that you
> **MUST NOT QUIT!**
> Jake Steinfeld

A heart rate monitor is an invaluable tool because you don't have to guess anymore – you'll know. I'll be covering why this is so important in Stage 3: Exercise. Don't miss it!

The fight against body fat is a real combination of efforts. For some examples of elimination, and of what works and what doesn't, please read on.

Example 1: one-out-of-three

You do strenuous cardio exercise a few times a week and come home to a nice bowl of pasta or rice, with absolutely no unhealthy fats. It's okay, but you're still not losing any weight.

Example 2: two-out-of-three

You do strenuous cardio exercises a few times a week and come home to a medium-sized serving of protein and a small serving of fibrous carbohydrates [broccoli, carrots, snow peas, etc], with absolutely no unhealthy fats. It's okay, but you're still losing only a little weight.

Example 3: three-out-of-three

You walk for 45–60 minutes a day, in your fat burning range for cardio, three to five times a week, and at night you eat a medium-sized serving of lean protein with a small serving of fibrous carbohydrates [broccoli, asparagus, green beans] and no unhealthy fats. You are finally losing weight – and it's not water or muscle, it's fat!

We've all heard it and we all know it. Now, what are we going to do about it? We need to address the real issues.

Reasons and excuses may give you something to talk about, but they won't give you the results you desire, Body & Soul. I have learned not to pull the 'time card' or the 'broke card' or the 'tomorrow card', because I value my life too much! We have ONE LIFE and every moment of every day matters. Let's nail these things once and for all!

LACK OF TIME

Probably one of the biggest and most common problems faced by most people is time – or lack thereof. It could be a genuine excuse or it may just be one that rolls off the tongue as easy as, "And an extra large fries with my double cheese and bacon burger, please!" Let's examine closely the excuses we have used to avoid getting in shape, whether they are valid or hilarious, and make a decision to make some changes.

LACK OF MONEY

If it's lack of money, then this book has certainly fixed at least part of that problem. Instead of having to pay anything from $50 to $150 or more per hour for your very own personal trainer – this book is an inexpensive yet worthwhile and highly valuable investment into your life.

PROCRASTINATION

If you have been battling for, say, five years and you now know that in less than a year, you could look and feel awesome, it would be a worthwhile investment of time, money and motivation.

A friend who has battled with 'bigness' all her life shared proudly with me that she is so glad that she started and finished. Her starting became her initial motivation, and the results from her efforts became her continuing motivation, until now, when she has far exceeded her original goals, because she decided she could!

TIREDNESS

There's more to it than meets the eye when it comes to taking good care of your body. It's much more than exercise, it's also good eating habits and plenty of rest as well. For some of us, it's also important to take time to relax and unwind, to alleviate the stresses of the day [I can certainly relate to this one].

Sometimes I look in the mirror at my face and think "yuk!", because all I can see when I look is that I haven't been taking care of myself. Whether from a lack of sleep, too many cups of tea or not enough exercise. That's when I take a grip and say, I'm going to do something about this – starting TODAY! Each of us requires different amounts of attention to function properly each day. Post-kids, I can get by with five to six hours sleep, although mostly my body craves eight or more hours. And some days, I have to have an afternoon nap because I can't think due to tiredness. This isn't good! And your body doesn't respond well to exercise when you are exhausted. The remedy is get more sleep!

YOUR PAST

One of the most common issues I face when helping people who are overweight is that there appears to be all manner of reasons for their physical condition. Be it an unhappy childhood, unhappy marriage, a traumatic event, or just pure 'genetics', there's always been something to take hold of and 'blame'.

Somewhere along the line, taking care of yourself has become the furthest priority from your mind, as the other issues and problems have crowded in around you. These issues and problems need to be released before you can move on. Please go through the process of establishing your enemies, and deal with these things once and for all. While you are not dealing with your internal pain, you are also not dealing with your external anguish. While you continue in your grief of soul, your body will also grieve.

NEGATIVE WORDS

Your enemies may actually be words that have been spoken over your life which have formed a frame in which you have been living. For instance, my friend who won her battle had always been a 'big girl', and had always been thought of and talked about as being 'big'. It was going to be difficult not only to change her physical shape, with the time and energy that goes into that, but also to bring about change in the opinions of others around her.

She had to be prepared to take up the challenge and win. She decided that nothing was going to be too difficult for her to change, because she really wanted the results that change would bring to her life. When we learn to turn our stress into strategy, we will change our lives.

SELF-DOUBT

Another great enemy is self-doubt and feelings of worthlessness. If you have no confidence in your ability to complete anything and don't feel worthy anyway, you don't stand much of a chance, now, do you?

You need to see yourself as you were created to be. If that means that we have to get below a few layers of 'winter coat', then let's begin that process slowly but surely. You are not alone. I understand what it is like to have tried and failed every diet and exercise program under the sun, and have met many other people who have failed as well. Whatever your body shaping enemy is or has been, be assured that it can be conquered.

HIDDEN ENEMIES

Are you aware of how much damage a Stealth Bomber can do in a war? Plenty! That's because you can't see it coming. The invisible enemy is probably the most dangerous. Go looking for those hidden things that will sabotage your progress!

> The thief comes only in order to
> steal and kill and destroy.
> I came that they may have and enjoy life,
> And have it in abundance
> [to the full, till it overflows].
> - Jesus
> John 10:10

Chapter

6

Body Types
and Metabolism

Slender, athletic, curvy and altogether beautiful.

There are three body types, and most people's lifestyles have led them to look like a mixture of two of them.

ECTOMORPH

An ectomorph has the body type that is most often seen in the pages of fashion magazines. They are slim boned, long-limbed, lithe, and have very little body fat and little muscle. Ectomorphs tend to have fragile, delicately built bodies and find it difficult to gain weight or add muscle. Supermodels, ballerinas and basketball players most commonly fall into this group. An ectomorph is naturally thin, can generally eat anything because of a naturally fast metabolism. Some ectomorphs may be underweight, but over-fat and thus be carrying too much body fat and not enough lean mass [muscle]. With age, even the super-fast metabolism of the ectomorph slows down and as a result, they often gain weight, since they are not used to exercising or watching their calorie intake. Even ectomorphs can't get away without exercise if it is a super sleek, toned body they are after.

Examples: Twiggy and Kate Moss

MESOMORPH

Mesomorphs could be thought of as the 'genetically gifted'. They are characterized by an athletic, strong, compact and naturally lean body. They have excellent posture. Often, their shoulders are wider than their hips and women tend to have an hourglass figure. Mesomorphs are natural born athletes and tend to be lean and muscular without trying. They generally are described as being of "medium" build. The world's leading tennis players, figure skaters and dancers fall into this group. Don't forget that most of us have a combination of two or more body types and therefore you may have some mesomorphic qualities! Although the mesomorph has a genetic head start, they tend to assume that they can get away with very little exercise. However, bad habits catch up with everyone in the end!

Examples: Gisele Bundchen and Sarah Jessica Parker

ENDOMORPH

Endomorphs have a soft, curvy and round physique and display the opposite characteristics from ectomorphs. They have a slower metabolism, gain weight more easily and have to work hard to lose body fat. Endomorphs often have a larger frame and tend to have wider hips than shoulders, creating a pear-shaped physique. Some of the most beautiful women in the world, though, are endomorphs.

Endomorphs will have a harder time losing weight. But it is absolutely not impossible to do so, but just understand that if you are an endomorph, you will have to work harder to lose the weight. Endomorphs do not have to be overweight. They simply require more determination than perhaps a mesomorph would, to achieve the same goal.

Examples: Marilyn Monroe and Beyonce

> Even if you were born with it,
> if you don't use it, you will lose it!

Ectomorph, mesomorph or endomorph... Which one [or combination of two] are you? Well, whichever one you are, it doesn't matter! There is a great body toning routine just for you! Initially, your body type and metabolism will determine where you start with everything. If you are an ectomorph or endomorph, you may not have as much natural get-up-and-go as a classic mesomorph, but you are able to work towards anything.

Then again, a mesomorph who is not at all athletically inclined, who would much prefer to watch basketball than play it, is going to be far less fit than an ectomorph who has been running marathons for the past five years. It's all relative when it comes to exercise. It's difficult for someone who was born an endomorph, and who has trained their way to being more of a mesomorph, to watch a classic mesomorph eating huge amounts of burgers and fries, never exercising, and looking exceptionally good, even at the age of 50!

The advantage that both the endomorph and ectomorph have over the mesomorph is the inbred ability and drive to do something to improve their body shape and fitness levels. It's called tenacity and it's a positive attribute.

This can work positively on their behalf to assist them to focus in other areas of life. Some mesomorphs don't grow up worrying about their physical condition, until one day all that bad eating and lack of exercise catches up with them.

For anyone who has been overweight for any significant period of time, life has been tough for you. The consuming and constraining anguish of each day rolls on, with the pressure that you have to do something about your weight. If this is you, you could start by stopping your thoughts about your size, and concentrating rather on your health.

> You have been created in the image of God!
> And you are approved of completely.
> Genesis 1 in the Amplified

Please don't instantly presume that you are naturally an endomorph just because you are trying to lose weight. Poor eating habits can push you into the 'hard-to-lose' category, but you may well be genetically one of the other types, or more likely a mixture.

The truth is that each body type is beautiful. When people are naturally curvy starve themselves to be a stick-figure, they have gone too far. We all need a revelation and understanding of who we are and what we are meant to look like [taking into consideration height, bone structure, etc], so we can set our body shaping goals accordingly. One is not better than another; each body shape is unique and beautiful.

Your metabolism is like an engine that constantly runs, keeping your body working, burning fuel for body functions and energy. It fluctuates throughout the day, depending on certain factors, including the time of day you eat and exercise.

You should eat larger meals in the earlier part of the day and smaller meals later in the day. This works with your body, rather than against it. It's a much easier method of losing weight and maintaining a long-term healthy lifestyle.

If your metabolism is slow from either genetics or poor eating habits, don't presume that it will never speed up. Some of the best success stories have come from people who have been overweight all of their lives, for both of the above reasons.

The great news is, in a very short time, no matter how long you have been overweight, you should be able to lose not only the weight you want to, but also expect that your metabolism will become faster and more efficient.

Without addressing the real problem of body fat, by trying diets here and there, you are virtually putting a bandage over a compounding problem. The only way to cure this problem is to naturally change your body's metabolism once and for all. It may mean you must have more diligence in the beginning, but you can increase your body's metabolism over time, which in the long-term will make life much more enjoyable for you.

I asked my Personal Trainer, Michelle Tolliver, to explain how our body's Base Metabolic Rate works:

"Your body has a Base Metabolic Rate that generally utilizes approximately 1000 calories per day, give or take a few hundred. The Base Metabolic Rate, or BMR, is the minimum amount of calories that your body burns to keep you alive. Any activity beyond this point will add to your total daily caloric expenditure. Your BMR can be increased through proper nutrition, and even further amplified by the building of muscle. Cardiovascular and weight bearing exercise will speed things up even further by stimulating your metabolism, and increasing your overall consumption of energy."

"With the knock-out combination of proper feeding, and even moderate exercise, you will observe your body instantly burning more fat, while sustaining a more stable energy level."

This book is written for everybody, which means it's for you. Whether you are a mesomorph who needs to become healthier on the inside and outside, or an ectomorph who needs to train for energy, or a mixture between the two!

All body types alike are always on the look-out for something that will work. Even an ectomorph can suffer from 'potbellyitis'. By the way, don't ever feel restricted by a definition, and remember your personal best! These definitions [endomorph, mesomorph and ectomorph] are just for your information, and not to make you feel bad about yourself.

I remember one of my clients was so thrilled to hear about this book, because he couldn't do any form of exercise as a result of injuries he's sustained during training of a period of years. When I got to the cause of the problem, I found that he had been running for fat loss and fitness, but he'd been running with injured shins, and continued to do so, until he basically couldn't walk. This is a great example of someone who not only didn't know their body, but didn't listen to it either.

In this case, short-term pain was not long-term gain. In fact, it was quite the opposite. At times we exercise madly in the hope that getting it over and done with quickly will make a difference in our lives. The reality is that this is very rarely the case. Once you know your body, you will come to realize that not everyone is born into exercise, nor do they need to be. We don't need a long history of sports involvement, and we don't even have to like it when we start. We do have to find a way of beginning and of nurturing our exercise habits, then the rest will take care of itself! You need to listen to your body. As you exercise, your body is constantly responding, telling you how you are progressing, and how well you are doing. Pay attention when your body tells you to slow down or stop.

Remember, an exercise program should be intended to make you feel healthy and well. It should not be used as an endurance contest, unless, of course, you want to be an elite athlete.

Speed Up Your Metabolism

Increasing your metabolism can help you burn calories and fat, while providing you with added energy. The key to increasing your metabolism is to understand what it is. Metabolism is a combination of physical and chemical processes, and together, these processes distribute nutrients that are absorbed into the blood after digestion.

Three factors determine your metabolic rate, which is the amount of calories your body uses every day. The basal metabolic rate [BMR] is the rate your body uses energy for vital body processes. The rate you burn energy during physical activity and the rate you use energy during digestion of food are the two other factors involved in your total metabolic rate. To improve your metabolic efficiency you need to alter what you eat and how active you are. Once you have done this, you will experience a difference in how you look and feel, Body & Soul.

The best way to jump-start your metabolism is to exercise. Exercise will reduce body fat and increase lean muscle mass. By increasing lean muscle mass, your metabolism will increase and aid in the weight-loss process. Muscle tissue uses more calories than fat tissue because it has a higher metabolic rate. Aerobic exercise, like walking, swimming or cycling, has the added bonus of speeding up your metabolism for 4 to 8 hours after you stop exercising. Additional calories will be burned off long after you stop exercising.

Weight lifting, resistance or strength training will also speed up your metabolism as it burns fat and increases your lean muscle mass, which increases your resting metabolic rate. A combination of aerobic exercise and resistance training is best for optimal fat burning and metabolism boosting. Exercise in the morning and you will reap the benefits of a faster metabolism throughout the day. By exercising just a little more than usual you can speed up your metabolism and use up stored fat in the process.

The good news is, you can jump-start a sluggish metabolism through exercise and diet, which will have lasting health benefits for you. Not only will you lose weight and gain muscle mass, but you'll have more energy to burn and you'll feel great, Body & Soul.

5 Keys to Body Shaping Success

1.   Focus your mind every morning on being a winner.

2.   Weigh what's on your mind as well as what's on your plate.

3.   Consider the effort required for your body to burn what you are about to eat. [1 hour walk = 300 calories]

4.   Crave freedom daily, way more than chocolate!

5.   Get back on track the very next day if you blow it!

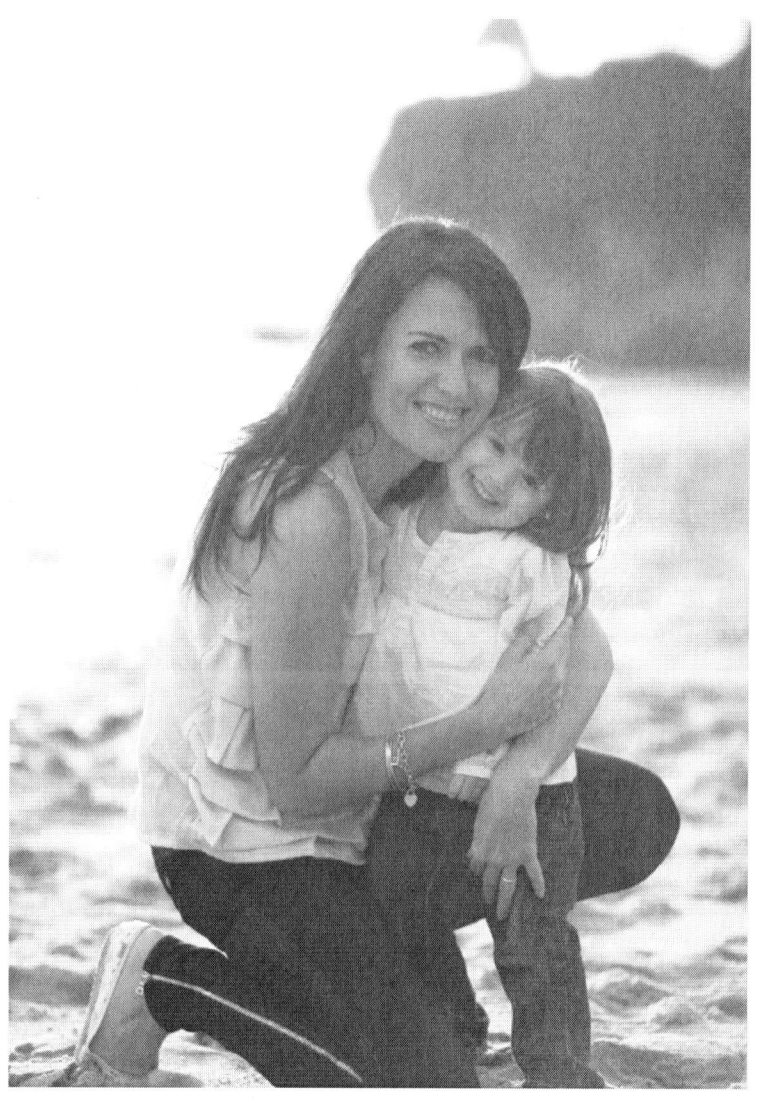

She is my motivation!

Chapter

Motivate Me

To provide with an incentive; move to action.

The average dieter stays on a diet for approximately three weeks – maximum. What happens after that? Usually, because they have deprived themselves so much, they end up eating far in excess of what they were eating before, just to balance what they have missed out on. Can you relate to this so far? We of good intentions!

That's normal for dieters on a calorie restrictive diet, but abnormal for you with your new Body & Soul Lifestyle.

GOAL SETTING

The key to getting this lifestyle to work for you is to establish goals and reach benchmarks. Your long-term goal, the end result, realistically may take some time, but to achieve your first short-term goal will only take approximately six to eight weeks. Later in this chapter, I've listed some easy steps to help you establish your long-term goal and to achieve your short and mid-term goals.

You need to set goals according to who you are, for instance, if you are naturally very curvy, don't set a goal to look like an ectomorph. That's impractical and will be de-motivating for you.

Your long-term body shaping goal will determine how many short and mid-term goals you need to set for yourself. Only set them one at a time, however, and remember when setting them that you are only human!

> Competing with others is sport.
> Competing with yourself is the true test.

The key for me has been to keep the goals short and sweet. I need to have a reason to walk for an hour a day. I make it a priority because it affects the rest of my life.

I need to know that once I have reached my short or mid-term goal, I am going out to dinner somewhere really special, or I'm buying some new clothes. It's only human to need to know you will receive a reward at the end of it all. Rewards are a great motivator!

The key to all this is that the reward should come from you. You arrange it and you deliver it, and know that you've done it for yourself and not because someone who'll never understand how hard it's been for you up until now tells you to do it. Achieving your new improved body shape possibly seems like a dream at this stage. Live the lifestyle and it will become reality for you.

To retain your new, improved body shape you will still need to be quite careful with your eating. The wonderful news is that your metabolism will be faster and you will be able to include a few more luxury indulgences every now and again. If you feel yourself slipping, though, you know how you reached your goal, and you simply need to go back to the beginning and reapply those same simple principles.

7 Keys to Effective Goal Setting, Body & Soul

1.   Have a vision – see who you want to become, daily.

2.   Know your strengths and your weaknesses and work with them, daily.

3.   Be completely honest with yourself, daily.

4.   Make sure your goals are achievable, daily.

5.   Find a way to exercise so that it is something you enjoy not endure.

6.   Live a life of action, daily.

7.   Focus on the freedom of your future.

It's important to remember too that a goal is more than a dream. It is a powerful part of your new Body & Soul Lifestyle.

Goals need objectives to make them tangible, so in setting your body shaping goals, be sure that you work on narrowing down broad thoughts so that they become objectives, and also be sure to turn thoughts of general intention into precise action.

Your goals should be like concrete, set in stone – similar to a tangible structure like a goal post on a football field. It's set there so you can cross over it and WIN!

GET A LIFE

The Body & Soul Lifestyle has been designed in every way to make getting into shape as efficient and easy as possible. This lifestyle is about losing bad habits and gaining a life!

You are being offered the 100% most efficient methods to reach your goals. Out of that 100%, it's really up to you just how much you decide to do. At least you will have a mark to measure yourself against – a check point – as far as effort you've put in, versus the results you've actually achieved.

If you put in 50% effort, you will gain 50% improvement, which may be all you want. You set the pace, and you choose. If your results aren't quite up to what you'd hoped for, then it's just a matter of taking on a few percent more effort. This is also a very good way to train an unwilling mind or body into doing what you want it to do.

This lifestyle is perfect for the busy person who wants to do as little as possible for maximum results. On its own, the nutritional section, [The Body & Soul Weight Loss Menu – Chapter 13, and The Body & Soul Goal Weight

Menu – Chapter 15], will give you wonderful results, enabling you to achieve a great deal more that you may have thought possible, and that's without even breaking into a sweat [yet!]

Having said that, it would be amiss of me not to encourage you to take on the '100%' Body & Soul Lifestyle, which will give you optimum results in the shortest amount of time [without cheating]. This of course includes some body shaping exercise – see Stage 3: Exercise.

Try and keep in the forefront of your mind why you started on this body shaping mission, and that too will help you keep on track. This may all seem overwhelming right now; but how long have you been unhappy with how you look and feel? It's time to bite the bullet and take action. The longer you think about it and wait for a miracle to drop out of the sky, the longer you are going to be unhappy. It's time to get practical and motivated to change.

It's truly amazing to see what I have seen in my business. People from all walks of life really have the same desires and needs as everyone else. Whether speaking for a large corporation, or some teenagers, or a small group of housewives and mothers, wanting to look and feel better is universal. You will be amazed at how many people will look to you for inspiration and support. This will also motivate and encourage you to maintain your new body shape. If you want to help others in the future, your pain can now help to become someone else's gain. It's amazing the kind of a fulfilling life you can build for yourself when your own personal healthy choices cause other people to be inspired by you.

When it comes to setting your goals, please remember to be realistic. It's the same principle as when you travel on vacation. You always tend to pack that outfit that you bought in a sale, in a rush, or that outfit that is two sizes too small that you somehow imagine will fit you better after a plane trip somewhere. Did you end up wearing those things? No! I know, because I've done this and so have you! We all think that vacation time is the golden opportunity to change habits, and get on top of all that we let snow us under every other month of the year.

The problem is that our goals for our vacation aren't realized and we end up coming home, not having worn all that stuff we packed, and not having finished one single book we brought with us, and in a sense feeling like we failed. It's the same with getting into shape. Why on earth say to yourself at 9pm on Sunday night, after eating a large pepperoni pizza by yourself, "I'm never eating pizza ever again." Get real! Of course you will, so it's a ridiculous statement to make. The same can be said of you desperately wanting to get in shape: "I'm going to start in the morning with my diet, and I'm joining the gym tomorrow afternoon and I'm going to do two hours of cardio and train in the gym all before I come home tomorrow night, and I'm going to do this eight days a week!"

It's more realistic if you haven't taken part in any exercise before, or for a long time, to start out slowly with a simple walking routine, maybe 30 minutes a day, two to three times each week, and then increase it. Remember though: results are directly reflected by the amount of effort you put in!

PERFECTION NOT REQUIRED

The definition of victory: saying you'll do something and actually doing it!

My main qualification for writing this book is that I do not have a perfect body! And I never will! "Hooray", I can hear you cheer! I am here to share some inspirational thoughts with you that will hopefully lead you to the revelation that there is no such thing as the perfect physique. Less than 2% of all bodies in the world resemble the supermodels we see adorning the pages of women's glamour magazines. This is not a real picture of what the women in the world look like.

There is a Greek word, 'Teleios', which interpreted means, ' perfect for now'. That is, perfect at our own particular stage of development. We all have a personal best, and that is what we are to strive towards.

It doesn't mean that we are to strive towards a supermodel body or an Academy Award winning physique, it means that we are to strive for our own personal best.

Has this thought released you? It certainly released me!

I believe that this is a great truth and a wonderful place from which to build a great new lifestyle. You can now look at yourself, and your own personal potential, and work within your own fence, and not the one across the 'supermodel' road.

Once you understand your personal best for now, you can watch it change and grow. 'Perfect for now' means that once you have read this book, and start to live your new lifestyle, you will become fitter and more toned, and your perfection or Teleios will also grow with you. It is an exciting process and really is without limitations!

I'm not one of those people who can claim
they love exercise.
But I do love all that it does for me!
Oprah Winfrey

I have found that at the core of most overweight people is a motivational thought that doesn't entirely revolve around themselves. Something I have found in common with many people I come into contact with is an eager desire to help others around them who are going through something that they can relate to.

For example, one of my clients who has battled with being overweight all of her life is a really lovely person, and continually talks to me about how she wants to change so that she can help and influence others to look after themselves.

I really encourage this type of outlook on life. It can only be a good thing. And it can often be the motivational point at which some people get themselves moving! To be able to do this, however, one must first become an example which others can actually follow.

Although I don't want to discourage anyone from helping others, it's important to be in a position of strength before you start trying to help others.

Victory is only sweet if you get to taste it. How do we have victory? By setting goals that are achievable, and then reaching them. Writing this book amidst a very busy life has meant that I have had to set goals to achieve my deadlines. The only problem with this though – and might I add that I am quite a disciplined person – was that I was setting goals that I had no way of achieving: walk for an hour, train at the gym for an hour, cook a gourmet healthy meal for my family, do five loads of laundry, take kids to and from school, feed and play with my baby, visit my neighbor, call my family, clean my house, iron my tea towels, help people, and then spend eight hours a day writing, 8 hours a day having coffees with people who need encouragement, spend some romantic time with my husband, and let's not forget to shower and blow-dry hair! Impossible!

I had to do some serious reality checks and change my goals for them to be realistic. Once I set goals for what was humanly possible [and I am known to push that limit from time to time!], then I began to experience victory in that particular area of my life.

It's the same with you. STOP setting unrealistic goals, and start experiencing victory!

A while back, it hit me suddenly that there is more to getting in shape than not being able to wear a mini-skirt for some women. If only it was a fashion problem – we could usher in the nice A-line skirt or bustle and train at will – but unfortunately the issue is far wider than this. I'm talking about thighs – you know, those pillars of strength that keep you standing, day in, day out!

A few years ago I was walking with a friend, someone who I never thought of as being overweight, although always looked solid. One day while we were walking she turned to me and said, "What's it like to walk without your legs rubbing together?" To be quite honest, until she posed this question, I'd never really thought about it!

Since that time, I have come across many women, who aren't necessarily all that overweight, who have struggled with the same issue. Also, after having kids, nothing is quite the same, and nor should be! Your tummy has just performed the miracle of its lifetime. I think it's amazing that it returns to any flattened shape at all. There are ways though, of reducing the *'squidge effect'*, through correct eating and exercise. It's much harder if you're a mamma who's had a taut little tummy, to find that only a few years later, you seem to have a little potbelly happening.

After four kids I can confidently say that it is possible for your tummy to be flat again. Just allow consistency to be one of your best friends! Living the Body & Soul Lifestyle, you will find great results in the stomach area of your body because most of the time, this problem area can be resolved with changing what and when you eat.

Now as for the back of those arms, what can I say? I know what I'm like. The slightest bit of weight on and I cover up for no-one to see! That's why I determine to stay in shape once I get in shape. I like to wear shorts and tank tops and I don't have time to worry about my arms, tummy or legs. Life's too short and I've worked too hard to achieve my goals and now I enjoy the freedom hard work brings!

THE TIME FACTOR

Time is something that if you feel you don't have, especially when it comes to looking after your physical well-being, you need to create. When I was on my Body & Soul mission to get back in shape after the birth of my daughter Bella, I discovered that if I was going to be able to get an hour's walk in every day, the only way I could do this so it didn't cut into the rest of my day was to get up at 5.45am and walk from 6am until 7am, from Monday to Friday. This is a very small sacrifice of an hour's sleep, compared to the wonderful benefits of getting fresh air, a fit heart, and great legs!

This time around, after the birth of my daughter London Eternity, I am able to walk a little later in the morning, but because of the time school starts for our teenage boys, I still get up at 5.45am! I love being a Mum!

Nothing in life is free, including our time. In fact, if someone tells me that they want something from me and it won't cost me any money, just a little of my time, every warning bell in me goes into mega-alarm. I truly do understand the issue of precious time. I also understand that precious time is useless time if we can't enjoy spending it! There is absolutely no use in working, working, working, if at some stage in your life, you don't stop and start enjoying all you've been working for.

If you are working too hard to stop and look after yourself, you need to sit down and prioritize your entire life. What use is it if you lose your life because of ill-health due to a pitiful diet and lack of exercise? It's time to sit back and think about what's really important. Life!

MONEY

You know, the whole money issue when it comes to exercise is something that need not be a problem. You don't have to join a gym, although if you can afford it, they are a great way of staying motivated, and all the equipment under the sun is there at your beck and call. If you have a roof over your head, some furniture in your house and can afford to buy a simple pair of dumbbells, you can have the body, health and longevity of your dreams.

Hey! And don't forget - walking is free! You don't need a $10,000 treadmill, you can walk around the block. Be creative and use what's available in your life right now.

And when it comes to the subject of eating healthy being expensive, it isn't so long as you stop eating junk!

FAMILY COMMITMENTS

Your family is so important, and time should be spent with them. It's really difficult to exercise when you have small children, but this is only for such a short time. Soon you will be on your way. I remember just before my twin boys were born, I decided that after their birth, I was going to work out at the gym three days a week, take them for a walk for an hour five days a week, and train clients when they were asleep during the day.

HUH! Talk about unrealistic goals! When my twin boys were born, I was in sheer survival mode. Forget exercise, I could hardly get out of bed to walk to the bathroom, I was so exhausted. I was feeding them every couple of hours and I was up and down with them day and night. Oh, the plans of mice and men!

It took a good six month period for me to even think about any kind of exercise. I had been so preoccupied with trying to get enough sleep that it's all I could think of for the first few months. When I did start, however, I was ready for it. My babies were a little older, and I started out slowly, and included them whenever I could when I walked. You can do plenty for your body by eating correctly, even if you can't exercise. But there is something that is irreplaceable – the invigorating feeling of exercise. Fresh air, deep breaths, worked muscles. Even if it takes some working up to, it's a worthwhile plan to include a realistic exercise routine in your life!

When London Eternity came along, I knew it would be my biggest body shaping challenge yet, so I made sure I planned out my life in such a way as to have plenty of time with my baby [I breastfed her for 16 months], and my other kids. I found myself wishing my body shape would change but I also found myself unable to set a proper time goal until after I stopped breastfeeding my baby. And because London Eternity is my last, I didn't know how I was going to do it, so I prayed that she would be the one to make the shift, and at 16 months she did! She was and is my priority, as are all of my kids, and my husband, of course!

We need to be in shape for our family, but we also need to make sure that we have plenty of time for them. Kids spell LOVE like this.... 'T I M E'.

7 Keys to a Establishing Your Long-term Goal

1. You must have a dream, so start to dream if you haven't already. Begin with the end in mind. Imagine the body you want to achieve. Put doubts out of your mind and keep focused on your plan.

2. Find a photograph of yourself or a magazine page which has a body shape you want to achieve on it, and stick it on your refrigerator door.

3. Tell one person you are doing the Body & Soul Lifestyle and keep yourself accountable to them.

4. Realize that what has taken you months or years to accumulate in size and, or habit, will take time and determination to lose and keep off.

5. Make a conscious decision that you aren't going to let your taste buds rule your life anymore.

6. Plan ahead, shop, cook and always be ready!

7. Think of all the people you will be able to influence and help, Body & Soul, when you have reached your goals.

7 Keys to a Starting Your First Week

1. Grab your favorite pair of jeans or a similar item of clothing that's one size too small, and choose one morning each week to try them on.

2. Measure yourself with a tape measure [or have someone else do it for you]. Always measure at the biggest point: shoulders, chest, waist, upper hips [including lower stomach], lower hips [including bottom and upper thighs], upper arm, upper thigh, calf.

3. Empty out your refrigerator and your pantry and don't store unhealthy food that will 'beckon' you to eat it!

4. Make sure you buy, prepare, cook and store lean protein and healthy foods so that you never run out.

5. Exercise as much as you can – ideally an hour's walk, 4-5 days each week is great, along with any time you can put in at the gym or at home doing weights.

6. Read your Bible every day and feed your spirit and soul with helpful positive thoughts, so that you can live the Body & Soul Lifestyle in faith!

7. Photograph yourself at the beginning and if you want to have your photograph taken weekly, make sure you wear the same clothes and be sure to be photographed in the place and same position. This will make the 'after' photos an exciting comparison!

7 Keys to a Reaching Your Short and Mid-Term Goals

1. The results you achieve will be your best motivation. Don't give up! You will be eating and sleeping better, you will have more energy, and people will notice how much better you're looking. You will have a glow about you that you just don't get with dieting.

2. Your new lifestyle of eating will be something you will be used to by now. As soon as you introduce added carbs and fats on your Treat Day, you'll really feel it!

3. It is important to consistently mix up your menu so that you don't become bored with your food choices.

4. If you have been walking most weeks, then mix up your exercise with some other cardio exercise, such as step machine, or elliptical.

5. Measure yourself with a tape measure even less often now. Try to do it just once a month. And, if you wish, jump on the scales – but remember muscle weighs three times more than fat! Don't be discouraged!

6. Grab the next article of clothing you want to fit into and keep it handy to try on once every two weeks.

7. Your clear skin and feeling of renewed energy will be something which will help you continue, and will also enable you to do more exercise.

Chapter

8

Commitment

Brave is commitment in plain clothes.

IMAGINE being brave enough to commit to changing your life. When we think of being BRAVE it is too easy to think of HEROES and automatically think we are not one of them.

My Dad was a fire fighter for 36 years. However, there was much more to my Dad's bravery than being a hero in an emergency. Being brave is all about courageous endurance. My Dad is a courageous man who has lived his life committed and consistent in his work, in his family and in his faith.

After the tragic events of 9/11 a New York Fire Chief was quoted to say...

"Fire fighters are going to get killed. When they join the department they face that fact. When a man becomes a fireman his greatest act of BRAVERY has been accomplished. What he does after that is all in the line of work. They are not thinking of getting killed when they go where death lurks. Fire fighters do not regard themselves as heroes because they do what the business requires."

> Brave is commitment in plain clothes.
> It isn't fancy promises and empty dreams.

There is a verse in the Bible, in Proverbs 31:10-14 that says, "She is like the merchant ships loaded with foodstuffs; she brings her household's food from a far [country]."

I love this verse because it suggests that our potential is enormous! We get to choose what kind of *vessel* we are going to be... *a merchant ship* or *a cruise ship.* We get to choose to take responsibility for our lives, or we can allow life to steam ahead over us. Maybe you feel more like a runabout boat or a dingy, or a ferry, just doing the same thing day in, day out, but God has designed and created you to be like a merchant ship for His purpose.

One thing to know about merchant ships is that they are not built in the ocean. Merchant ships are built in dry docks. Perhaps you are feeling like you are dry-docked in this season of your life. Take heart! That's exactly the best place for you to be when you want to change, rebuild and strengthen your life.

Whether you are sailing the oceans wide or you are being rebuilt in the dry dock, remember that God has designed and created you for purpose bigger and broader than you have imagined.

So what does that look like?

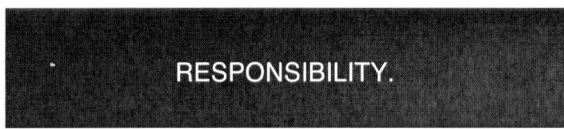

RESPONSIBILITY.

It means committing to being reliable and not random. It means committing to being responsible, and not a renegade. A renegade is a person who deserts a cause or a principle for something else. How often have you done that to yourself?

When we step up in our responsibility, we step down desertion in our lives. It means we become finishers, not quitters. It means we become fruitful, not futile. It means we become free, not imprisoned.

She or he who is brave is free.

Aristotle once said, "We become just by doing just acts, temperate by doing temperate acts, brave by doing brave acts."

Hey, it's easy to be brave from a safe distance, but brave is a doing word! Brave is all about enduring courage in the face of uncertainty.

There are shades of brave we all need to find. I found mine, now it's your turn to find yours.

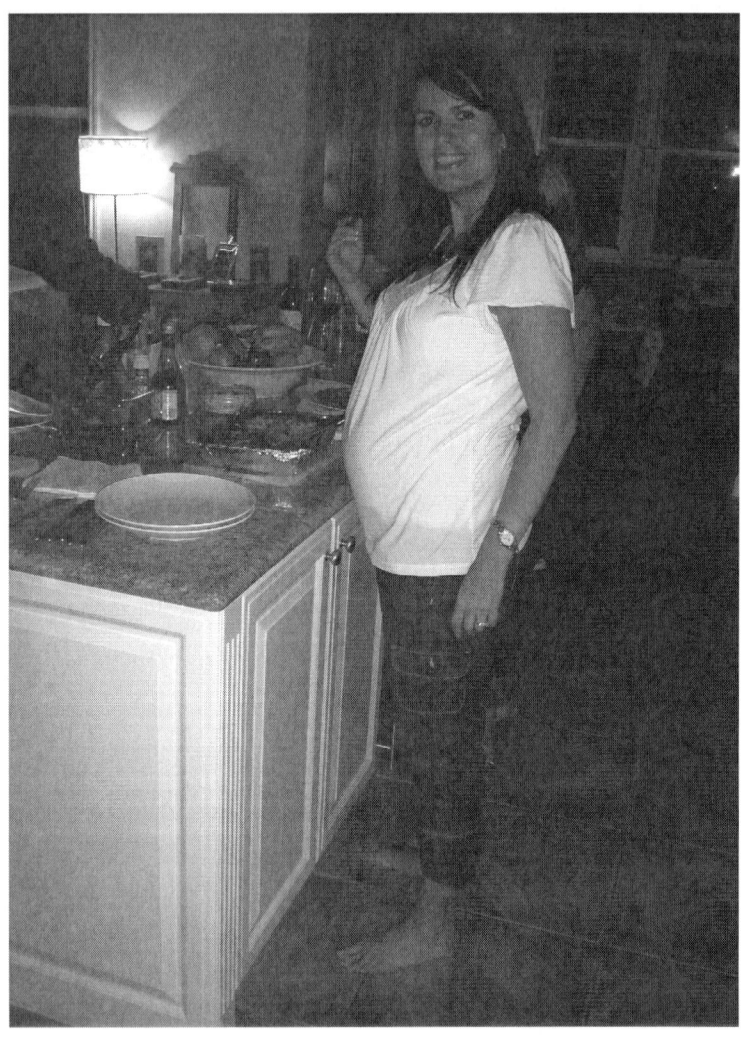

Here I am barefoot and pregnant in the kitchen…
And about to turn 40!

7 Keys to Commitment

1. Be committed to purpose.

2. Be committed to improving your health.

3. Be committed to create the life you want.

4. Be committed to being accountable.

5. Be committed to better relationships.

6. Be committed to change for good.

7. Be committed to freedom forever.

   "The Lord God is my Strength, my personal BRAVERY, and my invincible army; He makes my feet like hinds' feet and will make me to walk [not to stand still in terror, but to walk] and make [spiritual] progress upon my high places [of trouble, suffering, or responsibility]!"
Habakkuk 3:19

> I believe that two of the most important days in our lives are: .
> The day we were born and
> The day we found out why.

In the classic 1981 movie *Chariots of Fire*, the winner of the men's 400 meter race at the 1924 Olympic Games in Paris, Eric Liddell says an awesome thing…

"You came to see a race today. To see someone win. It happened to be me. But I want you to do more than just watch a race. I want you to take part in it. I want to compare faith to running in a race. It's hard. It requires concentration of will, energy of soul. You experience elation when the winner breaks the tape - especially if you've got a bet on it. But how long does that last? You go home. Maybe your dinner's burnt. Maybe you haven't got a job. So who am I to say, "Believe, have faith," in the face of life's realities? I would like to give you something more permanent, but I can only point the way. I have no formula for winning the race. Everyone runs in her own way, or his own way. And where does the power come from, to see the race to its end? From within. Jesus said, "Behold, the Kingdom of God is within you. If with all your hearts, you truly seek me, you shall ever surely find me." If you commit yourself to the love of Christ, then that is how you run a straight race.
I believe God made me for a purpose, but he also made me fast. And when I run I feel His pleasure."

I believe God made us for a purpose, but he also made us strong. And when we stand tall we feel His pleasure. I believe God made us for a purpose, but he also made us brave. And when we stop being afraid we feel His pleasure.

God has given each one of us the grace to be brave enough to commit.

Chapter

9

Consistency

Steadfast adherence to a particular course.

> Consistency is one of my best friends.
> Period.

When we decide to do something, there are many things or activities that will not give you the result you want in just one single action. For example, we cannot get an amazing body shape by just doing one session of exercise. We cannot be healthy by just eating one healthy meal. We will not have good relationships by just spending only day with someone and not staying in touch with them afterwards.

We cannot become wealthy by saving for just one day. We cannot become intelligent by learning for one day.

All these actions will need to be repeated on a regular, consistent basis until they create results. Unfortunately, many people stop working on themselves, body, soul and spirit, after a few attempts, thinking that the process will not work for them since they have already tried a couple of times. That is where the need for consistency kicks in. That is where we need to believe before we see. We need to understand the importance of consistency and harness its principle to our lives.

There are many businesses that were initially very successful after opening. They may have had many customers who admired what and how they provided either the quality of foods or their service. However, as time went by, perhaps the business owner started taking the initial success for granted, and therefore allowed standards to slip. Customers may notice the change and then stop frequenting the business.

Finally, those businesses are either closed down or sold to somebody else. This is due to lack of consistency. It is the same for a student who lacks consistency and needs to study hard near exam time. I think all of us know the importance of consistency but still we sometimes do not follow through and a lot of time throw off what we intend to do regularly. We always give ourselves reasons, most of which may be convincing, but completely futile.

Please don't let this happen to you! We need to create the habit of consistency in our lives.

Following are 5 keys to building consistency into our lives.

4 Keys to Consistency

1. Allow yourself to become irritated, uncomfortable and disturbed when you do not follow through. According to the principles of psychology, people do things either to avoid pain or gain pleasure. When you feel enough discomfort, you will make a change.

2. Stop rationalizing, quit making excuses. Even a good excuse won't get you where you want to go. We often give ourselves reasons for not following through.

3. Create achievable goal components. For example, how do you eat an elephant? One bite at a time! We can be more consistent with a long-term goal when we break it down into smaller daily components.

4. Always keep your goal in mind. Remind yourself what you will achieve by being consistent, and who else will benefit. Remind yourself of how you will look and how you will feel, once you achieve your goal. Regular visualization will stimulate your to follow through.

We can master our destiny by mastering our habit of being consistent on what we are doing. Consistency is also going to be a key element in creating a life in balance. Once we embark on any lifestyle change, it's important to make sure that all aspects of your life, in body, in soul and in spirit, are taken care of. And if you have a family, you look after them, too, as well as looking after yourself. The following are some keys to balance.

7 Keys to Balance

1. Decide what's really important. So many times we are overburdened in life because we take on everything that comes our way. Decide what's really important to you, and let the rest go.

2. Decide to focus on only a few things at a time. 3-5 is optimal and create ways you can add these things into your current routine.

3. Expect to mess up sometimes, and forgive yourself when you do. Get right back on track the next day/opportunity you have to be consistent.

4. Remember it takes some time to create a habit. Expect to spend at least 3 weeks to get on your feet.

5. Be flexible. Setting a routine is good, but realize life is not always perfect and you can still be consistent even if it doesn't look like you expected it to look.

6. Don't have a routine? Create a set of steps to do in a specific order every day. It will help turn actions into habits that you don't have to think about.

7. Be willing to adjust. You may realize after a week or so that something you thought was important really isn't. Be willing to drop the things that don't work, and fill that space with something else more important to you.

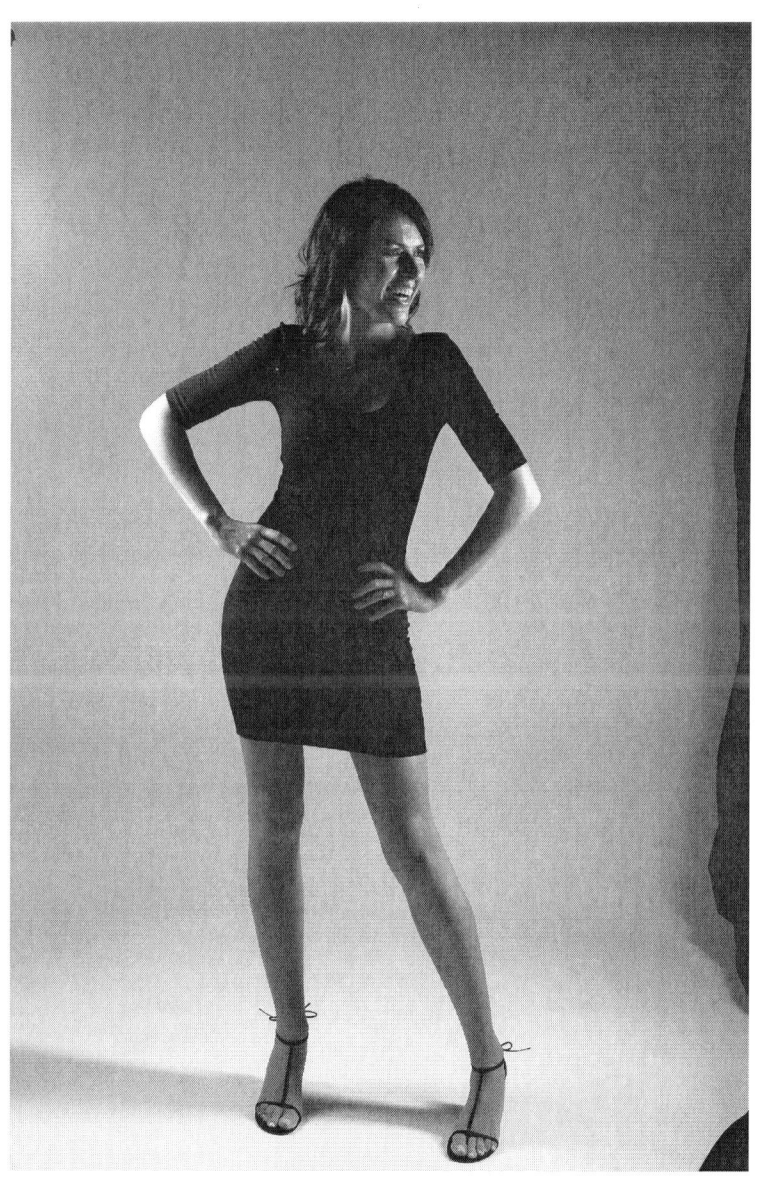

Be yourself, consistently.

It may be a good exercise to write down all the reasons you think you can't be consistent, and then come up with solutions beforehand so you are ready to combat the problems that might arise. Changing your mind will change your attitude, and changing your attitude will help change your life. Take it one day at a time. Don't worry that you might mess up next week. Concentrate on being consistent today and you'll be ahead of the game.

It's important to remove as many distractions as possible. And try to be as clear and specific with yourself with the things you know you need to be consistent in. Without a clear vision of where you want to be it's hard to move in the right direction.

Rewards come to those with consistent lives. Do what you can to make sure you don't bite off more than you can chew. Keep your changes small enough to be manageable - you're more likely to be successful if the thought of adding the item to your day doesn't completely overwhelm you. If it does, break it down into something a little smaller to start with.

If it's your goal to learn how to be consistent, then implementing even a couple of these tips will have you moving in the right direction.

Remember… Don't give up.

> … There should be a consistency
> that runs through us all.
> For Jesus doesn't change –
> yesterday, today, tomorrow,
> he's always totally Himself.
> Hebrews 13:7 in The Message

Stage

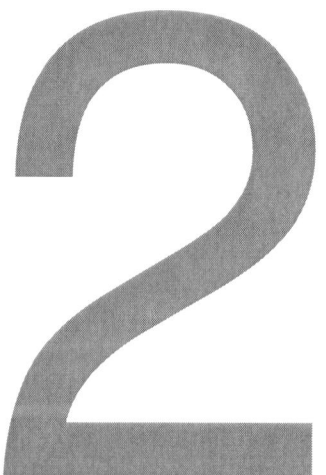

Food

Food

- ★ **Soul Food**
- ★ **Body Shaping Food Groups**
- ★ **Water and Other Drinks**
- ★ **Vitamins**
- ★ **Your Daily Menu Planner**
- ★ **Booster Menu**
- ★ **Treat Day!**
- ★ **Food FAQ**

Chapter

10

Soul Food

The emotional part of human nature.

One thing to remember the moment you decide not to eat the wrong kinds of food, is the moment that you will be tempted – sometimes beyond belief – to eat more of the wrong foods than you would ordinarily. That is because no-one likes deprivation. The moment we all tell ourselves, "No!" our flesh screams out, "Yes, yes, yes!", and it will always look for an excuse to win.

Every time stress hits your life you have a choice to go down the old road and fill your soul with comfort food, or you have a choice to put all that energy into carving out a brand new path. The difference between the old path and the new is vast. The old path had you worn out, Body &

Soul. But the new path will set you up to win, over and over again. We need to look up, step up and change! Take a look at the following 7 Keys to Strengthening Your Soul.

7 Keys to Strengthening Your Soul

1. Wake up!
Decide to have a good day.
> This is the day the LORD has made;
> We will rejoice and be glad in it.
Psalm 118:24

2. Look Up!
The best way to dress up is to put on a smile. A smile is an inexpensive way to improve your looks.
> The Lord does not look at the things man looks at. Man looks at outward appearance; but the Lord looks at the heart.
I Samuel 16:7

3. Listen Up!
Learn to listen. God gave us two ears and one mouth, so He must have meant for us to do twice as much listening as talking.
> Listen to advice, accept instruction and in the end, you will be wise.
Proverbs 19:20

4. **Stand Up!**

For what you believe in. Conviction is a powerful soul tool.

> *Let us not be weary in doing good; for at the proper time, we will reap a harvest if we do not give up. Therefore, as we have opportunity, let us do good...*
> Galatians 6:9-10

5. **Step Up!**

You can do it!

> *I can do everything through Christ who strengthens me.*
> Philippians 4:13

6. **Reach Up!**

For something higher.

> *Trust in the Lord with all your heart, and lean not on your own understanding. In all your ways, acknowledge Him, and He will direct your path.*
> Proverbs 3:5-6

7. **Pray Up!!...**

Give God praise and ask Him to help you with what you need.

> *Do not worry about anything; instead pray about everything.*
> Philippians 4:6

We should strengthen our soul at the same time as we work on strengthening our body. That means we need to make sure we feed our soul with the kind of food that will satisfy well beyond a quick fix, or single 'meal'. Our souls may crave chocolate, bread, pizza, fried chicken and mashed potatoes, pizza, apple pie and ice cream, but these things don't satisfy, body or soul. Our souls may crave 'comfort', but true comfort doesn't come from physical food.

Traditional comfort or comfort foods have a deeply rooted emotional appeal and we need to treat them as such. Remember, if the enemy knows we live by our *feelings* he will *feed* us everything we *feel* like. Not only will this stop us from reaching our body shaping goals, but it will also ensure that our soul stays miserable, without the change it so desperately longs for.

So why is it when the weather outside is frightful, and forecasters start talking about snow, we start thinking about warming our hearts by warming our bodies with rich comfort food? Because we live traditionally instead of intentionally.

People have their own individual definitions of what dishes, specifically, constitute comfort food. For me, the category includes warm pancakes, hot chocolate, cheesy pizza, roast dinner, warm rolls and I could go on! Whatever its specific flavor and texture, comfort food, like all food, is a sort of fuel. But it's not like gasoline, whose purpose is to propel movement. Comfort food is more like firewood; its purpose is to help us feel warm, sheltered, safe.

Beware! It may make you feel warm and fuzzy for a moment, but the consequences from eating it, especially on a daily basis, will do anything other than make you feel warm and fuzzy. Generally a lifestyle of comfort food leads to a lifestyle of misery.

It so important to fill any void you may have in your soul with the right kind of *food* and to realize that your soul needs emotional fuel and your body needs physical fuel, so you don't confuse the two. We get ourselves in trouble when we try to feed our soul with physical food, and we get ourselves in trouble when we try to feed our body by emotion or will power alone.

Maybe you are carrying an extra 10 pounds that you have wanted to lose for years, and no matter how often you've worked out, your weight has stayed constant. Switching to a non-fat salad dressing may not be enough for you – it could be that you need to cut out bagels too, especially if a bagel with cream cheese has been a lifeline comfort food for you.

Whether it's chocolate cupcakes, homemade lasagna, or a big packet of salty chips, we all have favorite foods that give us more than just calories! We crave certain foods because we associate them with pleasant memories, like family celebrations, or consider them rewards because that's how they were presented when we were young. That's why when we're sad or stressed we reach for cookies or muffins rather than chicken or celery.

The good news is that when weighing whether to indulge in comfort foods, it doesn't have to be all or nothing. You can enjoy them on your Treat Day, and when the time is right. I certainly found it easier not going there with 75 pounds to lose, until I was just about at goal weight. Whatever you do, remember comfort foods are for occasional indulgence and not something that should be part of your new Body & Soul Lifestyle every day.

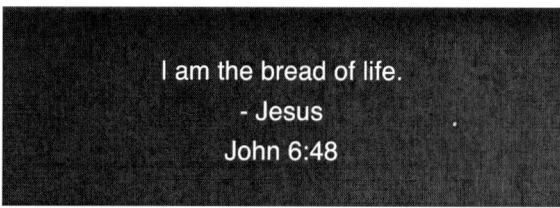

I am the bread of life.
- Jesus
John 6:48

Soul food was originally developed by enslaved African-Americans who lived under the difficult and impoverished conditions of grinding physical labor. It was humble, hearty food traditionally cooked and seasoned with pork products and often fried in lard. Traditionally, an important aspect of the preparation of soul food was the reuse of cooking lard. Because many cooks were too poor to throw out shortening that had already been used, they would pour the cooled liquid grease into a container. After cooling completely, the grease re-solidified and could be used again the next time the cook required lard. I can remember my Grandmother and Mother both re-using lard when making a roast dinner, and how incredible the vegetables [especially the potatoes] tasted.

The problem with frequent consumption high fat and high carbohydrate ' comfort' or ' soul' foods, without significant exercise is that they contribute to unusually high occurrences of obesity, hypertension, heart conditions, and/or type 2 diabetes. And these conditions, left untreated and unchanged, often result in shortened lifespan. Additionally, trans fats, which are used not only in comfort and soul foods, but in many baked goods, is a known contributor to cardiovascular disease. Don't eat it!

A great way to *feed* your soul, is to *feed* your mind with positive ideas. See the following list of 10 Keys to Feeding Your Soul *[while feeding your body]*.

10 Keys to Feeding Your Soul
[while feeding your body]

1. Think of yourself as being in shape, Body & Soul.

2. Plan your eating routine. Do not wait until you are hungry to plan a meal or snack.

3. When eating, take the time to enjoy your food. Do not watch TV or play on the computer while you are eating.

4. Sit down and eat, do not eat while standing up.

5. Converse during mealtime and take the time to enjoy food and fellowship at the table.

6. Set your fork down at least once during your meal and take a moment to reflect.

7. Chew slowly and be mindful of what you are eating and why.

8. Don't put more food on your plate than you are supposed to eat.

9. Don't go back for seconds.

10. Mealtime shouldn't be a race. Take your time to appreciate eating good food!

Chapter

11

Body Shaping Food Groups

A group of foods that have a common purpose.

This chapter has been designed to help you understand the different types of foods I'll be suggesting that you eat, and why. I've explained not only what to eat, but why and how it will affect your body shape.

If you don't particularly like the food I've suggested, or if you are allergic to it, it can, in most cases, be substituted. Once you read through all the detail, you should be able to create your own personal body shaping food pyramid.

There are many ways to lose weight but there are fewer ways to actually shape your body. There are certain foods that your body needs more of than others, and for a season, there will be certain foods that are best for you to eliminate completely.

> Food can be a means to an end, or it can be enjoyed. I say EAT intentionally… and ENJOY!

For me, chocolate is a dangerous item on the list. The reason chocolate is so dangerous for me is because once I start, 'it' [chocolate can talk!] tells me that I can't stop! So I very rarely have chocolate unless I am ready to engage in a 'conversation' of limitation!

PROTEIN

Protein is a vital part of your daily eating plan. It also happens to be one of the most misunderstood areas of nutrition. Meat farmers expound the virtues of the 'near-medicinal' qualities of various meats. Then there are the vegetarians, who propose life after hamburgers with lentils and soy beans. Finally there are the health fanatics, drinking shape-up shakes and miracle slimming drinks. So what is what, and who's right and who's wrong? These groups all have fairly sound reasons for their choice of protein intake. The Body & Soul Lifestyle goes a step further, however, to find out what is best for us in our quest for a better body shape.

Most people don't ask themselves why they are eating. If you are reading this book, I presume your reason is to change your body shape, so let's look at the options for eating, in that particular context.

Protein is your body's building blocks. If you took all the water out of your body, you would be left with just over 50% pure protein. Now that should give you something to think about. Your body also annually renews more than 95% of all its molecules, and every molecule is made up predominantly of protein and water. That's how important protein is!

Now, as impressive as that information may be, you still need to know how that relates to a better body shape. Unfortunately, most dieters forget this next very important point: muscle will only tone and shape if there is enough protein to feed it. The reason we want muscle to tone is so we will look and feel better, but even more importantly than that, is the fact that toned muscle is incredibly efficient at burning fat. Muscle uses fat as fuel, so the more toned and stronger your muscles are, the more efficient they are going to be at burning fat. For example, a 4-cylinder car doesn't burn very much fuel because the cylinders are small and it is not a very powerful vehicle, but an 8-cylinder vehicle needs many more gallons of fuel because it is much more powerful.

We are going to turn everyday movements and activities into fat and calorie consuming workouts!

This is why protein is so important!

In deciding which protein is best for you to eat, always choose leanest and freshest protein available.

MEAT PROTEINS

To help you better understand this section I am referring to meat proteins as any animal product, including poultry, fish and dairy products. Meat can be an excellent source of what are called 'complete proteins'. Protein is made up of amino acids, and 'complete proteins' contain all the eight essential amino acids in the quantities needed to be fully used by the body. If a food doesn't contain all the amino acids in the correct ratios, it is called an 'incomplete protein', because the body cannot use it.

You don't need to know in detail which amino acids do what, unless that is of particular interest to you. Then you should do some research! It is fairly easy to remember that all meats and dairy products have the eight essential amino acids in good amounts, and that all vegetables, fruits and grains either don't have any at all, or they are substantially lacking in them.

So from this perspective, meat proteins are a good choice. Of course, as you will read on the protein guide, some meats are much better than others because of their fat content. Generally, fish and white meat are going to be better for your body shaping endeavors, and so should be considered before all others when choosing a protein from this category.

VEGETABLE PROTEINS

As already mentioned, vegetables are not great sources of protein on their own. When it comes to consuming enough to meet your daily requirements, this can cause a problem – especially if you are exercising or are fairly active. To ensure you are getting the complete eight essential amino acids from vegetables, dried beans, peas, lentils and grains, you must eat two or more of these foods together, for example, dried beans and a grain such as brown rice or couscous.

Being a vegetarian can turn into a science of its own, learning what goes with what. At the end of the day, vegetarians will often still have consumed under the optimum daily requirements, because of the low amount of essential amino acids – gram for gram – in vegetables.

Most people know that nuts and soy beans are relatively good forms of protein. However, they are both proteins that are not readily absorbed by the body, and nuts contain large amounts of fat! So eat them raw and eat them sparingly!

'SLIMMING' SHAKES

This is an interesting area where, unfortunately, what may seem a good idea, can grow into a 'monster'. Have you ever read the contents on the labels of some of these drinks? You could become slimmer drinking a melted chocolate sundae because some are so high in sugar! It is, however, very easy to distinguish the good from the not so good, and it is well worth the effort to do so.

Protein shakes are actually your BEST option for optimum body shaping results. Providing you have selected the correct type, they can be a wonderful source of protein and much lower in fat than meat. Again, if you select the right type of protein powder, it will be far more easily absorbed by your body than meat or vegetable protein. And another good reason is that protein drinks are convenient, filling and relatively inexpensive.

What you should be looking for is either whey protein isolate or whey [being basically the only ingredient], egg albumen and casein. They are all low in fat and high in protein. It's important to read all the ingredients on the labels, because if the shakes contain sugars, full cream, vegetable or any other oil, give them a big fat miss! Those containing soy protein too high on the list of ingredients are selling you a little short of useful ingredients.

IN SUMMARY

Armed with the protein guide, you should be able to make the best choices every time, now knowing the importance of choosing wisely. One last thing to remember: it doesn't matter how fabulously high in amino acids and how absorbable or low in cholesterol the protein is if you cover it in fat when cooking it.

Remember: all meat should be unprocessed, that is, fillets only. Cooking should be done as low fat as possible – just a little olive oil is okay. Use a non-stick pan, grill, barbeque, or oven. Steam, char-grill, bake and ENJOY!

Hey!
Think before you buy.
Think before you cook.
Thank God before you eat.

PROTEIN

LEAN PROTEIN

WHEY PROTEIN ISOLATE PROTEIN SHAKE:

These are the best form of protein available at present. Although available as one of many ingredients in a few different types of protein powders, the best form is when it's basically the only ingredient. WPI is the most highly absorbable protein available and is less than 1% fat. It is convenient as you can mix it and take it to work, and mix it in cooking if you wish. The latest scientific evidence shows that whey protein concentrate can actually boost the body's immunity by up to 500%. It's a great natural appetite suppressant and contains properties which help speed the body's metabolism. But it's important to understand that WPI is not a meal replacement, or a protein replacement; it is a natural protein. Consider it as a piece of chicken, for example, and have it with a small salad for dinner.

However, it's most important that you do not confuse pure WPI with ion exchange or ionized whey protein. There are some protein supplements available which contain these ' high tech' ingredients, which unfortunately have undergone a considerable amount of chemical treatment. This treatment removes much of the valuable calcium, as well as many of the other beneficial properties of pure WPI, including the immune boosting and cellular regeneration benefits. Pure WPI is not chemically treated, and the protein structure remains as nature intended it, ready for our bodies to be nourished by it.

EGG ALBUMEN PROTEIN SHAKE

This is another good form of protein. It is available in a powder mix and is fairly inexpensive. It is very absorbable and low in fat. It too is convenient, as you can mix it and take it with you to work; also you can use it in cooking if you wish.

EGGS

Eggs are a great form of protein – there is absolutely no cholesterol in the whites, which is what I recommend you eat most of. Only have up to two yolks per day. One egg yolk scrambled with four egg whites in an omelet is delicious. Simply mix with some vegetables and use a non-stick frypan. Eggs are inexpensive and should be used often in your eating plan. In case you are wondering what to do with the unused yolks – feed them to your pet!

WHITE FISH

By white fish, I'm referring to fresh fish that isn't canned, and it's also not tuna or salmon. It also isn't other types of seafood. White fish is very good for you, it contains a minimal amount of fish oil and is excellent grilled or baked just using a little olive oil. Don't batter and fry as that will defeat the purpose of eating this wonderful lean protein.

Some examples of white fish are: halibut, whiting, sole, perch, cod, sea bass, etc. Always make sure you buy fish from a reliable source so that you know it is fresh, and be certain to store properly in a refrigerator so that the fish doesn't spoil before cooking.

DARK FISH

Dark fish is tuna and salmon, and any other type of fish that has dark flesh. It usually is a little oilier than white fish. It is, however, an excellent source of protein and is readily available – especially canned tuna and salmon, if you are unable to buy the fresh variety.

Tuna contains the least amount of fat of the brown fish varieties. Remember, when selecting any tinned food, go for tuna in brine or spring water, not in oil. Some of the new varieties of tuna snacks available contain oil and mayonnaise, so be careful. Most of the tinned salmon is very oily, so purchase freshly filleted salmon when possible. Pink salmon is fractionally lower in fat than red salmon. We eat a lot of fresh grilled salmon in our home because it is readily available and tastes amazing, and is so good for you!

TURKEY

Turkey doesn't have to be saved for Christmas dinner – it is lower in fat than chicken! Turkey is a wonderful source of protein and you can cook it in the same way as you do chicken. You can also substitute it for the chicken in any of the chicken recipes. Try to stay away from processed turkey as it may be high in fat and most probably loaded with sodium. Fresh is always best!

CHICKEN

Chicken seems to be a universally popular form of protein, loved by most adults and kids alike. Chicken is easy to cook in a variety of ways, and it's great to eat hot or cold. Make sure that you eat mainly chicken breast, as the thighs, legs and wings contain a higher fat content. Also, ensure that all traces of skin, fat and gristle are removed before cooking. Again, try to stay away from processed chicken. Remember, the way you cook your chicken will determine how many calories you will end up eating.

VEAL

When you're buying veal, make sure to ask your butcher if it is tender, and then ask him to trim off any fat. You will usually have to trim again at home, as most butchers don't think that 'that tiny bit of fat' will hurt you. We know it will! Cook it slowly and carefully.

BEEF

Beef is high in protein, essential vitamins and minerals, including iron, but you do only need a small piece of it now and again. Include it in your weekly eating plan for variety and taste, but please limit it, because it's number nine on the list, which means there are eight other leaner, lower in fat types of protein to go for first.

LAMB

Lamb is quite high in fat, even when it's lean. It's only included here for a change in scenery. Lean filleted lamb is delicious marinated with sweet chili sauce and chargrilled. Have a look at the Roast Lamb with rosemary recipe – it is amazing. Look out for Australian and New Zealand lamb as it is the best in the world!

PORK

Again, I've added pork here but only for variety. It is now available much leaner than in years gone by, but even in its new, lean form, it is really still too high in fat to eat on a regular basis. Only buy the pork fillets and make sure you go over the meat for any traces of fat before cooking.

VEGETABLES

If you are a vegetarian and you don't eat any dairy products or eggs, then your choice of protein is limited. A combination of vegetables will get you where you want to go, if it's your only choice, but just watch the fat content of what you're eating. You can combine green veggies with grains and rice, or mushrooms with green peas, brussels sprouts, broccoli and cauliflower, or soy beans with brown rice or wheat. Remember though, there is no protein in fruit. Try to include whey protein and eggs in your daily eating plan.

FATTY PROTEIN

[Listed from bad to worst]
Grams of fat per 100 gram serving, ie - % of fat]

•	Bacon [grilled]	19.2
•	Soy beans [dry]	20.2
•	Sausages [thick]	21.3
•	Roast pork [2 slices]	26.7
•	Lamb chump chop [fatty]	28.0
•	Salami	33.9
•	Pepperoni	36.0
•	Spam	30.6
•	Peanuts, dry roasted	47.6
•	Sunflower seeds	51.3
•	Pine nuts	71.0

Fatty protein should be left out completely, including all kinds of processed meats. Fresh and lean is always best!

CARBOHYDRATES

Carbohydrates [carbs] were thought to be fattening until not so long ago. The first thing a dieter would do is drop potatoes, pasta and bread completely from their diet. This, of course, left little of any substance to eat, and so left the poor dieter starving!

Then came the carbs revolution: "They are okay." The experts said they have little or no fat, and a new form of dieting was found. So then, why isn't everyone trim and taut as promised? After all, carbs don't have fats unless you add them, do they? Let's see why.

The main role of carbs in the body is as an energy source. Without them, you'd barely be able to do normal day-to-day tasks, let alone try to maintain a healthy exercise regime as well. The body specifically uses carbs when it's working anaerobically [without oxygen]. For example, carbs are like fuel for people who like to really 'huff and puff' throughout a workout. Unfortunately, that's where the problem with carbs lies.

The modern dieter, who takes in plenty of low-fat carbs morning, noon and night, had better be busting a gut for hours on end to ensure all this excess fuel is burnt up. Otherwise it will be stored as FAT! Wouldn't you rather be busting your gut burning fat instead of carbs? [More later!]

One myth ripe for dispelling is that eating a lot of carbs will give you heaps of energy, as the advertisements for breakfast cereals would have us believe. Unless you are fit and toned, it's like putting premium fuel into an old car. It won't really add to the performance until the engine has been tuned. And, unlike the car, we get another top-up each day, so our fuel tanks have to expand to take all the excess.

There are several different types of carbs, but we are mainly concerned with fibrous and starchy. Starchy carbs are digested much quicker than fibrous carbs [crunchy vegetables and bran] so they instill a higher concentration of energy into the blood. That's why you are told to eat a banana when playing sports. Unfortunately though, if your body cannot burn the energy there and then, it stores it.

Check out the following carbohydrate guide for the different types of starchy and fibrous carbs. Although carb foods don't contain much fat, the body is easily able to convert them into fat for storage, if they are not used.

However, carbs do play a vital role in the Body & Soul Lifestyle. Below is the good news about carbohydrates.

5 Good Reasons to Eat Carbs

1. They reassure your body that you are not in a famine, inhibiting the slowing of your metabolism.

2. They help to fill you up if eaten in moderation.

3. They contain vital vitamins and minerals.

4. They help provide energy for good training and energetic living.

5. They contain most of the roughage required in your diet.

As you can see, carbs are a powerful weapon for healthy living, but must be eaten wisely.

The best way to enjoy the benefits of carbs has been explained in Body Types and Metabolism [Chapter 6].

Starchy and fibrous carbs are known as complex carbohydrates. Another carbohydrate is sugar carbs, known as simple carbohydrates. Simple carbohydrates are usually refined or processed food, as opposed to the more raw or unprocessed complex carbohydrates. They are digested very quickly into the system, and release large amounts of glucose into the body – hence the sugar rush from eating a chocolate bar.

The problem with simple carbs is that you must burn them off with exercise, or else they will be stored!
Fibrous carbs are a vital part of any diet, as well as healthy living. Fortunately, fibrous carbs can be eaten all day, in filling amounts, thus aiding good internal health on your way to a great external shape.

Although in the following carbohydrate guide I have referred to amounts of each starchy carbohydrate to eat each day, this is only a suggestion. You will be the best judge of what your body needs each day. If you find that your results are too slow, maybe it's time to cut back a little more on your starchy carb intake. It's impossible to prescribe exactly what you need, as everyone is different. You will become the best judge in time.

CARBOHYDRATES

STARCHY CARBOHYRATES

These are important in your daily eating plan. The amounts you eat and the time of day you eat them will help determine your body's shape. And remember, while you are wanting to lose weight, you will need to limit these and once you have reached your goal, you can introduce them slowly and enjoy in moderation.

Pay now by limiting them, and play later by enjoying them, and the benefits of what that will do for you.

CEREAL

Your breakfast shouldn't be wasted on eating cardboard – no matter how low in fat the cardboard is! You should eat something which is high in fiber and filling, such as oats made with skim milk, or some other high fiber and low in fat and sugar cereal. If you have a favorite low-fat cereal that happens to be high in sugar, use it just as a topping over your more healthy cereal. Be careful: even though some cereals, including muesli, low fat, these figures are provided on a very small amount and they are possibly very high in carbohydrates. You have to make choices which will help determine your body shape, so read the packets and be wary.

PASTA

Nearly everyone eats pasta. It can be enjoyed in many different ways – although for a great body shape, I suggest you steer away from traditional Italian dishes loaded with olive oil. Make up your own recipes, or check out the variety listed in the Body & Soul Recipes section. Limit your intake of pasta though, as it does take a substantial amount of activity to use it all up. If pasta is part of your lunch, eat around half a cup of cooked pasta, maximum. Pasta encompasses all different types of noodles, including instant. Be wary of the two-minute noodles that are coated in oil. Go for the low fat variety instead.

RICE

Rice is easy to cook and is great with any meat or veggies. Although brown rice is fractionally higher in fat than white rice, it is a better choice. It has more fiber, is more difficult for your body to absorb, and more likely to be burned off. If you really cannot stand anything but white rice, then eat it. It's more important that you choose what you will actually stick to. There are some great fragrant rices on the market, such as jasmine. Remember, you don't need a lot for energy – a little will take you a long way. Don't forget, even rice noodles, although low in fat, are considered starchy carbohydrates.

POTATOES

You are probably thinking, "What's dinner with no potatoes?" It's a better body shape – that's what it is! Although low in fat themselves, potatoes are starchy and stored easily by the body unless you are quite active.

Jacket potatoes cooked in a hot oven without oil are great, or jammed with finely chopped veggies and strips of charbroiled chicken breast. Eat and enjoy them, but just make sure you limit them! If you were having them for your lunch, only have one medium-sized, or a couple of smaller-sized potatoes.

BREAD

We've been told in recent times that bread is fine, it's just what you put on it that's potentially not! That's true enough, but too much bread can make a difference when you're trying hard to get into shape. Limit your bread intake to around two pieces per day. Go for the normal-sized bread, not the super-duper-can't-fit-in-the-toaster sized bread. Wholegrain breads contain more fiber and, similarly to brown rice, are going to aid in speeding up your metabolism. If you must eat white bread, go for the newer variety of white bread which is very high in fiber. Bread includes anything made of flour – muffins, scones, pastries, rolls, pancakes, waffles, etc.

FIBROUS CARBOHYRATES

FRUIT

You can eat any fruit, but limit bananas as they are fairly high in sugars and carbs, and avocadoes, which although low in cholesterol, are really high in fat. You'd need to train like an Olympic athlete before burning them off! Eat a couple of pieces of fruit each day, but try not to have any at night, when your metabolism is working at its slowest.

Stay away from fruit juices, even if they are 100% fruit, because they are very high in fruit sugars. A diluted glass once in a while is okay, but certainly not daily. Water is always your staple drink for a great body.

Also, limit your intake of dried fruits because you tend to eat more of them. Certainly don't get caught thinking that dry mixes from the health food shop are going to be good for you. They are loaded with nuts, natural sugars and fat.

VEGETABLES

All veggies are great. When you know what your starchy carbs are, you will become more inventive with your fibrous carbs. Vegetables such as carrots, celery, cucumber, green beans and lettuce can literally be grazed on all day. When eaten with plenty of water throughout the day, they actually work as 'negative vegetables', meaning they burn more calories and fat than they contain themselves! They're excellent for snack attacks. Try to only lightly cook your veggies. The crunchier they are, the more fat they can help you burn. And if you are going to add a little oil, make sure it is olive oil.

FATS

Fats are very misunderstood.

Like most other areas of nutrition, scientists discover something new about fats on a regular basis. However, we need to be sure that we have the best information available with regards to fats, because what we do with them will make an enormous difference to our body's shape.

Let's look at the three types of fats.

Saturated Fats

Are really bad heart attack material. These are dripping, lard, butter, and vegetable oil.

Polyunsaturated Fats

Are low in cholesterol, and sold to make you feel good! They contain the same nine calories per gram as saturated fats. These are most margarines, even light, low, cholesterol free ones.

Monounsaturated Fats

Are sold as healthy, until you start trying to believe that you won't actually get fat from eating fat – wrong! They also contain the same nine calories per gram as saturated and polyunsaturated fats. These are olive oils.

What's good about fat?

The body needs fat for protection of its organs. It also needs fat as an energy source for aerobic activity. At this point, I'd like to explain the difference between aerobic and anaerobic activity, so you can better understand the fat-burning process.

Aerobic Activity

Believe it or not, aerobic activity is not jumping around in an aerobics class at your local gym, nearly killing yourself because of the lack of oxygen your body is suffering from. It is steady exercise, such as walking or cycling. As a result of taking part in steady aerobic exercise each day, your body will burn fat.

Anaerobic Activity

This is the type of activity that has caused many people to give up exercising completely. It should be left to the fitness fanatic. Most people are not fit enough to benefit from taking part in high-impact aerobics or spin classes. There will be more on this very interesting topic in the Exercise section [see Stage 3]. When you are breathless, your body is unable to burn fat, as it requires oxygen to do the job!

To be healthy, it is important that your body contains some fat. But take a good look in the mirror. It probably looks as though your fat stores won't run out for a while! Having said that, if you have an eating disorder, or if you have a tendency to see yourself as fat when everyone around you tells you that you are not, be very careful. Reducing your calorie and fat intake when you are underweight can cause serious health problems. If you're unsure, ask your doctor.

The Weight Loss Menu Planner [Chapter 13] and Goal Weight Menu Planner [Chapter 15] contain plenty of fat, most of which is unseen. By unseen fat, I mean fat in an egg yolk, fat in skim milk, fat in low-fat yogurt, a splash of olive oil in a salad or when cooking, fat in really lean meat, and fat in fish oil, from fish. This amount of fat is plenty to live on, so don't be surprised when I say you should positively, absolutely, not add any more! This is what sets the Body & Soul Lifestyle apart from any other 'diet' around.

DAIRY PRODUCTS

Dairy products are in a category of their own because they contain a good mix of the three other categories: proteins, carbohydrates and fats. They can be the best in protein and the worst in fat!

So many people have given up dairy products because they believe doing so will make them healthy, and it seems almost trendy to do so at the moment. Lactose intolerance has become a catch phrase. Unfortunately, though, a great number of people are cutting out dairy products for no real reason.

Low-fat dairy products are God's gift to a great body shape – and nothing short of! A low-fat, sugarless yogurt can make your day much more bearable when you crave junk food, and can be eaten any time of day.

Because of the high-fat content of cheese, it's best avoided. Unless it is around 98–99% fat free, even the low-fat brands contain more than a desirable level of fat.

Always read labels carefully and if you must eat a cheese, choose wisely and eat in strict moderation.

Skim milk can be turned into a fruit smoothie delight. It too can be consumed any time of day. It is a great protein and very low in carbohydrate and fat.

If you feel that you are, or may be, lactose intolerant, try taking in small amounts of dairy products [with the okay from your doctor first, of course], as this may slowly stimulate the enzymes you need to tolerate lactose in your body.

Chapter

12

Water and Other Drinks

Liquid essential for life.

Most of us are aware that we should drink water. Few people, however, realize how vitally important it is to our well-being. To give you some idea of how much water is contained in your body, have a look at these statistics:

Lungs:	90%
Blood:	82%
Brain:	76%
Bones:	25%

Many people suffer from lethargy and tiredness in the afternoon. However, in nine out of ten cases, it's not sugar or carbohydrate energy that's lacking, it's the effects of dehydration.

Water is best absorbed by your body plain, or with some fresh lemon or lime juice added. Drinks such as tea, coffee and alcohol actually cause dehydration, so the more of these you drink, the more water you should consume. For example, for every cup of tea I drink, I try to have two extra cups of water on top of my daily water requirements.

What are the daily water requirements? Current wisdom says eight glasses a day – but how big is a glass? I am recommending that you drink at least one and a half liters of [preferably bottled or filtered] water each day. If you're not sure of this amount, keep a used drink bottle, wash it and refill it each morning.

You'll be surprised how easy it is when it becomes part of your daily routine. The more water you drink, the more thirsty for water you become.

Flavored drinks can't be considered plain water, as flavored liquids will often be digested differently. Add a squeeze of fresh lemon or lime juice if you need flavor. Remember, some flavored drinks can dehydrate you, so be sure you reach your one and a half liter quota of plain water each day, minimum.

Tap water these days is far from beneficial to your health – especially if you are drinking several liters of it. The chemicals which are added to clean it are quite toxic, and too many of them can be cumulative.

Sports drinks are very over-rated, and one of the big traps for body shapers. Stick to water instead.

Good intentions can lead to the consumption of several hundred calories you simply do not need. If you are overdoing getting fit, or training for an event, then a fluid replacer, or electrolyte can help. But if you are burning fat at optimum levels, then water is more than adequate for re-hydration.

Alcohol is high in carbs and calories and is best kept for Treat Days, in moderation of course.

If you feel that you can't get enough energy for the early-morning walk, a cup of coffee or tea with non-fat milk will give you a boost.

For a pick-me-up, diet colas are another form of caffeine that you can drink if you wish. I don't recommend you go crazy with these drinks. And the super turbo charged energy and vitamin drinks aren't great to drink on a regular basis. Drink them sparingly.

Water is the best option, each and every time. Around 80-100 oz per day is what you should drink.

Chapter

13

Vitamins and Other Supplements

Something added to make up for a deficiency.

So often we hear people say, "I get all the vitamins I need from food". The unfortunate reality is that this is extremely unlikely for the average person because of pollution, toxins, fast living, stress, lack of exercise, over-exercise, or simply because of the poor nutrients in the food most people eat.

Most processed, mass-produced food is treated, refined, stored, preserved, irradiated, frozen, force-fed, chemically enhanced, and/or grown in industrially polluted farm soils with cheap, nutritionally empty fertilizers that produce a lot of empty, water-filled produce.

Sounds appetizing, doesn't it? Just one of these factors is more than enough to ruin the nutritional quality of food, and if it doesn't, there is always the way we cook and store the food at home that will really finish off the job!

Although it is suggested that you eat plenty of fresh fruit, vegetables, dairy products and lean meats, it's important to realize that even the freshest of foods are often subject to inadequate growing, storage and handling these days.

So, to prevent illness and to ensure maximum health and performance of your body [and that includes your ability to burn fat and shape up], I suggest a few simple vitamins to include daily.

VITAMIN C

Vitamin C is vital for the production of collagen, which is the cement that binds just about your whole body. An antioxidant, it helps to build the immune system and protects against free radicals that cause old age, as well as helping to repair the body after a hard day. The minimum amount taken per day should be 1000 to 2000 mg. An orange contains 10 mg of vitamin C, so you can see how many of them you'd have to eat! If you feel run down or as though you may be coming down with something, double the dose, or even triple it. It's important that you take vitamin C before you get sick, as it works far better as a preventative medicine than it does a cure.

VITAMIN B COMPLEX

Vitamin B complex is the commando of the B group of vitamins. It's great against stress, and when used properly, it can aid in inhibiting fatigue. Remember that Vitamin B in a tablet form can only be absorbed sublingually [dissolved slowly under the tongue] or in an advanced form of an injection, by a medical practitioner. Be sure to follow dosing instructions on the label, as doses can vary greatly between manufacturers.

MULTIVITAMINS

It is very important to purchase a good-quality multivitamin. A lot of vitamins can be bought quite cheaply, but what most people don't realize is that in the case of vitamins you really do get what you pay for. The cheaper vitamins are usually the least absorbable and in very low doses, so you need to take more. Go for quality, as this ensures that you are not missing anything important in your diet. Ask at your local health food shop or drugstore if you aren't sure about what's best for you.

FIBER

Not all fiber supplements are created equally. There are three main types of soluble fiber supplements: psyllium, methylcellulose, and polycarbophil. Each type of fiber has varying uses, side effects, and properties. Talk with your doctor about fiber supplements to determine which is best for your body. When shopping for fiber, look closely at the ingredients to discover which type of fiber is used in each commercial brand. Be sure to rule out fibers with added sugars. Remember to start at a low dose and drink plenty of water.

CALCIUM

Calcium is a vital mineral. Many women, and nearly as many men, are calcium deficient, and don't even make the minimum recommended daily allowance! The so-called calcium-rich dairy products contain calcium that is only about 20% absorbable. The 800 mg recommended daily allowance that you think you are getting from your two glasses of full-cream milk is only giving you 170–200 mg of useable calcium, which leaves you 600 mg short. Again, be aware that many calcium supplements are not well absorbed and therefore are a waste of money. Calcium carbonate is the most absorbable.

IRON

Many people - especially women - are iron deficient. This is another example of poor modern living. An iron supplement is essential, if you are indeed deficient. Iron is responsible for carrying oxygen in the blood, so you can see that since the brain and muscles need oxygen to work, iron is vital. Coffee and tea can actually block the absorption, so this is another great reason to supplement your iron intake.

Chapter

14

Weight Loss
Menu Planner

Reduction of body fat for improved Body & Soul.

The different foods listed on the following pages are simply suggestions that have worked well for me. If you can find suitable alternatives, go right ahead, but remember to watch the fat content of anything you include. Keep the amounts medium-sized at first. If you feel you're not getting the results fast enough, cut back a little. If you feel as though you could eat a horse at the end of the day, then increase a little. It's important to find your own balance – it's a personal thing.

When you are cooking, use either non-stick pans or good quality stainless steel pans, and remember to use olive oil sparingly when cooking. And really watch the amount of starchy carbs you eat each day.

TIMING YOUR MEALS

Your body's energy levels vary throughout the day. Rather than depriving your body of necessary foods that may be considered heavy, such as starchy carbohydrates, the following is a schedule which enables you to eat plenty of nutritious foods, although probably in a different order than what has been normal for you.

This is an area of habit replacement which will prove vital to improving your body's shape. Making correct choices will give you the results you're after.

In the following pages of your Weight Loss Menu Planner, you'll see that at the top of each page is a box containing essential information about the type of food you should be eating at that meal and the time of day you should eat it.

It's important to understand that your Weight Loss Menu Planner has been designed to help you lose weight, so use my guidelines, but feel free to adapt them to your lifestyle. So you know the boundaries: you cannot change the type of food to eat at each meal, but you can change the timings within a half-hour flexibility radius.

This means that if it's 11.30am and you haven't had your mid-morning snack, then make sure you still eat it – but have it before noon. Then, because you're running a little late, have your lunch at the later end of the scale, and get back on track ready for your afternoon snack.

Once you learn this lifestyle, it's easy. Your body actually does the learning and remembering for you. It will let you know that it needs a meal or a snack, and when you check your watch, you'll realize that it always lets you know right on time.

DURATION OF THE WEIGHT LOSS PLAN

The following Weight Loss Menu Planner is suitable for you to use [providing you have your Doctor's permission], for 8 weeks maximum. If you still want to lose more weight beyond the 8 week mark, then you will need to follow the Goal Weight Menu Planner in Chapter 15 for 2 weeks, so that your body has a chance to stabilize, prior to your next phase of weight loss.

After those 2 weeks, you are able to embark on up to another 8 weeks using the Weight Loss Menu Planner. If you want to lose more weight, then you'll need to follow the Goal Weight Menu Planner in Chapter 15 for another 2 weeks.

And so the cycle continues, depending on how much weight you want to lose. If you don't break the routine after 8 weeks, the Weight Loss Menu Planner will no longer continue to work, as your body will become accustomed to it, and it may even begin to store body fat. And no-one wants that to happen!

Slowly and surely wins the race. Don't be in so much of a hurry that you try to cut corners, because those corners actually become foundational pillars in your life that will help you stay in shape in the future.

Work hard and be at peace Body & Soul.

WEIGHT LOSS MENU PLANNER

Breakfast
Any time you wake up and are ready to eat!

1 piece of wholegrain toast <u>or</u> 1/3 cup of oatmeal
1 egg

Start with 8oz of water, then you can have tea or coffee with your breakfast. Don't drink any fruit juice as it's high in sugar. You will not necessarily feel full after eating this meal.

Your mid-morning snack is just around the corner, so pace yourself and you will be full enough in time.

Breakfast kick-starts your metabolism for the day and will help in burning fat and raising blood-sugar levels, increasing your general energy.

WEIGHT LOSS MENU PLANNER

Morning Snack
Approximately 2 hours after breakfast

1 protein shake or 1 small non-fat sugar free yogurt
Then 30 minutes later
1 apple or other high fiber fruit

Drink 8oz water first, then you can have tea or coffee with your snack. If you like, you can have a diet soft drink instead of the tea or coffee, but not instead of the water, and preferably not every day!

After a couple of days, you will crave this snack. It's part of breakfast and part of lunch. It puts you into grazing mode, which keeps your metabolism on fire, and this helps again in burning fat.

The most amazing part of this snack is that if you miss it, by 5 or 6pm, you will know it! If you have cravings at that time of day, which is normal for most people, it's because you have missed this snack, or your afternoon snack.

WEIGHT LOSS MENU PLANNER

Lunch
Approximately 2 hours after morning snack

4oz fish or lean meat
1 cup fibrous vegetables, e.g. broccoli
2 cups dark green lettuce
salad dressing [1 tablespoon olive oil max]
fresh lemon, squeezed

Drink 8oz water first, then eat.

Your lunch will become the focus of your day, just as your dinner has been in the past, as it is now the main meal of the day.

Make the absolute most of this meal, because for the rest of the day the meals become smaller and smaller!

WEIGHT LOSS MENU PLANNER

Afternoon Snack
Approximately 2 hours after lunch

1 protein shake or 1 small non-fat sugar free yoghurt
Then 30 minutes later
1 apple or other high fiber fruit

Drink 8oz water first, then you can have tea or coffee with your snack. If you like, you can have a diet soft drink instead of the tea or coffee, but not instead of the water, and preferably not every day!

Again, after a couple of days, you will actually crave this meal. It's part of lunch and part of dinner, in the grazing mode. If you miss this important meal, you will definitely feel it around 6 to 8pm!

WEIGHT LOSS MENU PLANNER

Stop!
Hold it right there!

Please read this before you go any further...

Because your body's metabolism slows down later in the day so you can sleep at night, the later in the day you eat, the more careful you must become in your selection of food.

To help you, dinner has been split into two sections, depending on whether you eat early or late.

WEIGHT LOSS MENU PLANNER

Early Dinner
[5pm to 6.30pm]

4oz fish or lean meat
1 cup fibrous vegetables, e.g. asparagus
2 cups dark green lettuce
salad dressing [1 tablespoon olive oil max]
fresh lemon squeezed

Drink 8oz water first, then eat.

The earlier you eat this meal the better. For absolutely optimum results in the shortest amount of time [without cheating], you can have a protein shake and salad for dinner each night, whether it's early or late. Try it and see how you do. Take a break for a couple of weeks and try it again. You will definitely like the results!

Ensure you go for variety, and don't let yourself become bored! Save the dessert recipes listed in the Body & Soul Recipes section for your Treat Day.

WEIGHT LOSS MENU PLANNER

Late Dinner
[7pm or later]

3oz to 4oz fish or lean meat and ½ cup of vegetables
or
1 protein shake

What you eat for this meal is crucial. Again, for absolutely optimum results in the shortest amount of time [without cheating], have the protein shake as your first choice. The great thing about the protein shake is that you can mix it in the morning and take it with you if you are going to be out late – and you don't have to think twice about what to eat for this important meal.

If you're prone to the midnight munchies, relax – this will go away. Try a cup of hot lemon water, until your body gets used to your new routine.

If you really need more food, have a protein shake before bed.

Chapter

15

Booster Menu

What to do when you reach a state or level of little or no progress.

If you are doing everything right and you are not seeing the results you feel you should, it could be that your body is 'stuck' in a plateau. If you've ever tried to lose fat for any sustained period of time - you may have hit a plateau. You have changed nothing, but suddenly the fat no longer disappears. The human body is incredibly adaptive, and will do its level best to maintain equilibrium [homeostasis].

The plateau effect has to be the biggest motivation-killer there is. The best single word of advice is to make a change. Don't make the mistake of doing the same thing over and over expecting a different result.

Booster Menu

BREAKFAST: 1 egg
                          And half a grapefruit

MORNING SNACK: 1 protein shake

LUNCH: 3oz white fish
                          And half a cup of cooked spinach
                          with fresh lemon juice
                          And half a grapefruit

AFTERNOON
SNACK: 1 protein shake

DINNER: 3oz white fish
                          And half a cup of cooked spinach
                          with fresh lemon juice
                          And half a grapefruit

SUPPER: 1 cup hot water with half a lemon
                          boiled in water for 3 minutes.

Plateau usually happens because your body arrives at a weight that it has been before. It's super important for you not to give up. We'll mix up the menu slightly, for just 2-3 days, to get things moving again.

Don't give up!
All your efforts are money in the bank.

Chapter

16

Goal Weight Menu Planner

The achievement toward which effort is aimed.

Once you have reached your goal weight and size, it's important that you stay on track, otherwise you will quickly undo all your hard working efforts. Your body needs to create a new 'set-point' and that means you will need to be very careful not to gain anymore than 2-3 pounds for the next six months, minimum. The good news is that you are now able to eat more and as long as you continue to exercise regularly, you should find this stage relatively easy.

Remember again the time and effort required to get you to your goal and stay focused. You have fought for freedom and won and now is not the time to kiss it all goodbye by overindulging too soon and too much.

To avoid regaining weight [or not gaining extra weight in the first place], the energy your body burns off must equal the energy you take in from food. To achieve this it is essential that you feed yourself exactly the same amount of calories as your body burns off. In this way, there will be no surplus calories left over to be stored as extra weight. But, how can you guess this amount of calories? In order to balance your calories, you need to work with specific numbers.

The balance between the number of calories coming into your body and the number of calories your body burns off is known as your energy balance. Controlling your energy balance is like controlling your bank account. If you ignore looking at the specific numbers in your bank account and just try to guess that the money coming into your account equals the money going out...well, do you see the problem? And yet, this is how millions of people attempt to manage their weight every day!

Knowledge is very important. You need to know what you're eating, how many calories the food you consume contains, and you need to know how much energy you are expending every day. This may sound like a lot of work but trust me, it is far less work than living the 'yo-yo' lifestyle every day, not knowing if you'll be up or down. Once you know what you're doing and it becomes a lifestyle for you, it is so simple and really then boils down to choice. You may know that something is going to tip you over the edge but you want to eat it anyway, because you know you will be extra careful for the next few days. That's freedom of choice. Where you lose your freedom is *presuming* you'll be ok without knowing you're ok.

After six to twelve months of being within 2-3 pounds of your goal weight, you can slowly introduce other foods that you enjoy, and you can certainly enjoy Treat Day once every week. Again, if you gain 5 pounds or more, you will need to go back to the weight loss menu planner and do it until you get back on track.

Try as hard as you possibly can to not go above the 5 pound mark. Just as it is for weight loss, it is for weight gain...

> If I can gain 5 pounds, I can gain 10
> If I can gain 10 pounds, I can gain 20.
> If I can gain 20 pounds, I can gain anything!

Scary thought, but true!

You have the tools you need now, so get on track, stay on track and don't trade that freedom you've fought for, for anything!

I believe in you!

Breakfast
Any time you wake up and are ready to eat!

1 piece of wholegrain toast or 1/3 cup of oatmeal
2 eggs

Start with 8oz of water, then you can have tea or coffee with your breakfast. Don't drink any fruit juice as it's high in sugar. You will not necessarily feel full after eating this meal.

Your mid-morning snack is just around the corner, so pace yourself and you will be full enough in time.

Breakfast kick-starts your metabolism for the day and will help in burning fat and raising blood-sugar levels, increasing your overall energy.

GOAL WEIGHT MENU PLANNER

Morning Snack
Approximately 2 hours after breakfast

1 protein shake or 1 small non-fat sugar free yoghurt
Then 30 minutes later
1 apple or other high fiber fruit

Drink 8oz water first, then you can have tea or coffee with your snack. If you like, you can have a diet soft drink instead of the tea or coffee, but not instead of the water, and preferably not every day!

After a couple of days, you will crave this snack. It's part of breakfast and part of lunch. It puts you into grazing mode, which keeps your metabolism on fire, and this helps again in burning fat.

The most amazing part of this snack is that if you miss it, by 5 or 6pm, you will know it! If you have cravings at that time of day, which is normal for most people, it's because you have missed this snack, or your afternoon snack.

GOAL WEIGHT MENU PLANNER

Lunch
Approximately 2 hours after morning snack

5oz to 7oz fish or lean meat
[gradually start with 5oz and build to 7oz
over two weeks]
1 cup fibrous vegetables, e.g. broccoli
2 cups dark green lettuce
salad dressing [1 tablespoon olive oil max]
½ cup brown rice or 1 slice wholegrain bread

Drink 8oz water first, then eat.

Your lunch will become the focus of your day, just as your dinner has been in the past, as it is now the main meal of the day.

Make the absolute most of this meal, because for the rest of the day the meals become smaller and smaller!

GOAL WEIGHT MENU PLANNER

Afternoon Snack
Approximately 2 hours after lunch

1 protein shake or 1 small non-fat sugar free yogurt
Then 30 minutes later
1 apple or other high fiber fruit

Drink 8oz water first, then you can have tea or coffee with your snack. If you like, you can have a diet soft drink instead of the tea or coffee, but not instead of the water, and preferably not every day!

Again, after a couple of days, you will actually crave this meal. It's part of lunch and part of dinner, in the grazing mode. If you miss this important meal, you will definitely feel it around 6 to 8pm!

Stop!
Hold it right here [again]!

Please read this before you go any further...

Because your body's metabolism slows down later in the day so you can sleep at night, the later in the day you eat, the more careful you must become in your selection of food.

To help you, dinner has been split into two sections, depending on whether you eat early or late.

GOAL WEIGHT MENU PLANNER

Early Dinner
[5pm to 6.30pm]

5oz to 7oz fish or lean meat
[gradually start with 5oz and build to 7oz
over two weeks]
1 cup fibrous vegetables, e.g. asparagus
2 cups dark green lettuce
salad dressing [1 tablespoon olive oil max]
½ cup brown rice or 1 slice wholegrain bread
[if you are carb sensitive and feel that your body doesn't
need more carbs at night, you can eliminate the
rice/bread at night]

Drink 8oz water first, then eat.

The earlier you eat this meal, the better. For absolutely
optimum results in the shortest amount of time [without
cheating], you can have a protein shake and salad for
dinner each night, whether it's early or late. Try it and see
how you go. Have a break for a couple of weeks and try it
again. You will definitely like the results!

Ensure you go for variety, and don't let yourself become
bored! Save the dessert recipes listed in the Body & Soul
Recipes section for your Treat Day.

GOAL WEIGHT MENU PLANNER

Late Dinner
[7pm or later]

5oz-7oz fish or lean meat and ½ cup of vegetables
or
1 protein shake

What you eat for this meal is crucial. Again, for absolutely optimum results in the shortest amount of time [without cheating], have the protein shake as your first choice. The great thing with the protein shake is that you can mix it in the morning and take it with you if you are going to be out late – and you don't have to think twice about what to eat for this important meal.

If you're prone to the midnight munchies, relax – this will go away. Try a cup of hot lemon water, until your body gets used to your new routine.

If you really need more food, have a protein shake before bed.

Chapter

17

Treat Day!

Anything that affords particular pleasure or enjoyment.

THE DAY YOU'VE BEEN WAITING FOR!

For being so very good and sticking with the Body & Soul Lifestyle, you can have one Treat Day each week – maximum.

Treat Day should start once you have reached your goal. You can have a Treat Day every week while you are trying to lose weight, if it makes it easier for you. Personally I find it easier to introduce Treat Day after I have reached my goal. Treat Day means you can have a little indulgence one day each week. Please note though that it is **TREAT DAY** and not **TREATS DAY!** There is a big difference and you need to stay focused!

One tip though...
I STRONGLY SUGGEST THAT YOU TRY TO
KEEP TREAT DAY TO ONE MEAL PER WEEK.
That is if you want the best results ...
which I know you do!
ENJOY!

With all the hard work that goes with healthier eating, the Body & Soul Lifestyle provides you with some release. It's TREAT DAY, one day per week. Having a Treat Day each week not only keeps you sane and makes the days in each week pass quickly for you, but it actually aids in speeding up your metabolism.

The body doesn't know what's happening when you eat fat after not eating it all week, so your metabolism goes into overdrive. It works in your favour to have a Treat Day once a week, providing, of course, you go straight back to the Body & Soul Lifestyle the next day!

There's obviously varying degrees of damage you can do on your Treat Day. You will find that you don't have to go all out to become satisfied. A little goes a long way, especially when your body is not used to eating junk anymore! When you reach your body shaping goal, you will be able to have more than one Treat Day a week, without making any difference to your body shape. That's the benefit of having a faster metabolism and learning to live a disciplined lifestyle – forever!

Chapter

18

Food FAQ

An expression of inquiry that invites or calls for a reply.

WHAT ABOUT CELLULITE?

Cellulite is fatty deposits in the body, and not toxins blocking fat, or anything else. The only way to get rid of cellulite is to get rid of the fat, by eating properly and exercising. You can do this by following the Body & Soul Lifestyle. It all comes down to what you eat, when you eat it, and how much exercise you do. There is no magic lotion or potion to eliminate cellulite. Genetics also have a part to play, and that can mean that cellulite is either easy or more difficult to get rid of for you. I had it, and I got rid of it by following the Body & Soul Lifestyle.

WHAT ABOUT SUGAR?

Sugar is something to be very aware of. Look for it and don't eat it! It is found in most processed foods and in most 'health' foods. Although sugar does not contain fat, if it's not burned it will be stored as fat, so use it in moderation. Don't have it in your tea and coffee. Sugar substitutes such as artificial sweeteners or honey are alternatives, but eat them in moderation as well. Be careful to read the labels on everything. Sugar and fat together can be a disastrous body shaping combination!

WHAT ABOUT SALT?

Salt won't make you fat or thin, but it can aid in fluid retention. Because it contains no calories, and of course no fat, salt is helpful [in moderation] to use in cooking. If you have high blood pressure or a medical condition of concern to your Doctor, be sure to follow your Doctor's instructions.

WHAT ABOUT CHOCOLATE?

Chocolate contains carbs and fat. And, don't be fooled – carob is just as bad. So, save it for Treat Day. One tip though: if you have a sweet tooth and crave something, go for a couple of jelly beans instead of chocolate; at least they don't contain fat. If you are really craving sugar, especially later in the day, this is usually because you haven't eaten enough earlier. Have a protein treat and it will help take away the craving.

WHAT ABOUT PREGNANCY?

It's important that you don't do anything radical when pregnant. Take it from someone who knows. You need to eat plenty of fresh foods, but there is absolutely no reason why you shouldn't follow the Body & Soul lifestyle. Just be sure to discuss with your doctor. I found it incredibly hard to exercise throughout my pregnancy, but I do recommend you try to walk every day. You'll need this added energy when Junior comes along – believe me!

WHAT ABOUT BREASTFEEDING?

Even the head lactation consultant at the hospital advised me that I only needed to drink water to produce breast milk. Providing you are eating plenty of dairy products [low-fat, of course], and lots of fresh fruit, vegetables, grains, eggs and lean meat, not only will your doctor be satisfied with what you're doing, but you and your baby will be, too. Just keep coming back to the principles of the Body & Soul Lifestyle. I found that I didn't lose much of my weight during breastfeeding – it seemed easier to lose weight afterwards.

WHEN IS THE BEST TIME FOR TREAT DAY?

This is a personal thing, depending on your lifestyle. I enjoy having my Treat Day on the weekend, so I can enjoy my time off. If you find that because of circumstances, you need to have two Treat Days in one week, then just be extra careful for the following ten days or so. You know the principles and you know the balance.

My husband and I love to go out for Date Night on Saturday nights for an early dinner at our favorite Italian seafood restaurant. Enjoy whatever you want, but stay away from the bread that will be set on the table in front of you. If you have a choice, it's better to have Treat Day for lunch or early dinner, rather than eating late. At least then, your body has the rest of the afternoon or evening to metabolize it, well before you go to sleep at night. Number one rule though, ENJOY your Treat Day!

Stage

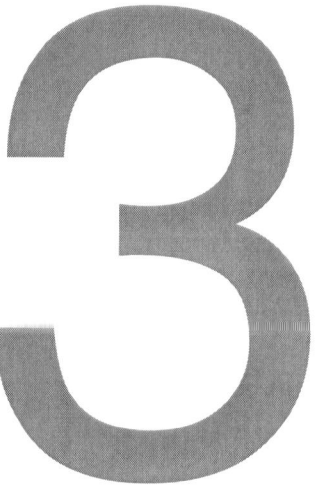

Exercise

Exercise

★   **Shape That Mind**

★   **Shape That Body**

★   **Start Today**

★   **Fat Burning Cardio**

★   **Muscle Toning and Strengthening**

★   **Zero In**

★   **Exercise FAQ**

Chapter

19

Shape
That Mind

To be firm in one's intentions, opinions, or plans.

Strengthen your mind and your body will follow.

What your body can do depends on what your mind can
conceive. It's all like a camera. Whatever the lens

captures, the film prints. We can't expect to produce a photo of something that has not been captured by the lens. The body needs the mind to imagine its potential.

When our mind is strong, our body will follow suit. When the mind is creative, the body will create accordingly. When the reverse happens, inability sets in. When the mind is weak and overwhelmed, the body takes over and commands the mind. Thus, at the slightest hint of difficulty and pain, the body will give up and tell the mind it can do no more. We all know what that feels like! Failure!

When the body doesn't feel like doing anything, for example, when you feel lazy and any excuse will do for not getting out of bed, and your mind is too weak to oppose your lazy thoughts, you have a case where your body leads your mind. Your mind is best used out in front!

Our mind is located in our head and our head is located at the top of our body. That is a visual picture of its leadership position in our life. Our body needs to be lead by a strong healthy mind. Many experts say a healthy mind always opts for a positive course of action, and very rarely inaction.

Once the mind decides something the body is unwilling to do, a tug-of-war starts. It is in such conflict that the body must be disciplined to succumb to the mind. If this is accomplished, the mind is strengthened and given authority over the body, which is trained to respond positively to its authority. The body does what it is told to do. So the body begins to outdo itself as the mind imagines it to be doing so.

Our mind and heart are linked so closely it is difficult to define them on their own, especially when it comes to decisions of our will. We need to pursue a healthy mind and a healthy heart. And we do this by reading God's Word

– the Bible, by believing what it says, and by acting on its clear and wonderfully uncomplicated instruction for our lives.

> You're blessed when you get your inside world
> – your mind and heart –
> put right.
> Then you can see God in the outside world.
> Matthew 5:8 in The Message

When our heart and soul are strengthened through our relationship with God, we gain so much more from life, Body & Soul. Everything changes, including and especially our attitude. Our attitude can make or break us. It's virtually indisputable that our attitude will determine how far we'll go in life. We need to recognize that a positive mental outlook can help us achieve optimal success, Body & Soul.

Having a positive mental attitude helps us cope with challenges. When we're put to the test, we're more likely to find inner strength to overcome adversity, and that strength just might be our winning attitude, which we have developed through strengthening our heart and mind in God. Whether or not we have all the tools, skills, knowledge, resource, or experience, our attitude can get us through tough times and come out on top.

On the other hand, an attitude filled with negative overtones makes everything much harder. You can't win when you go into a contest prepared to lose! If you expect to do well, your attitude will create positive, winning thoughts that help you succeed.

It's important to realize that for every effect in our lives, there's a specific cause. Through positive thoughts, we can control these causes and change effects or outcomes. In order to change your future for the better, you must first alter your thoughts in the present.

For every positive seed you plant, your thoughts will grow and reward you with a positive harvest. Negative seeds have the opposite effect. They'll grow, but result in a harvest of negativity. You can't plant negative seeds in your mind and expect positive results. It just doesn't work that way.

A vivid and defining difference between people who are successful and those who aren't is the way they think. Successful people visualize their goals and take action to make them happen.

Unsuccessful people dwell on the negative, spend their time and energy complaining, and worry about things that are unimportant. This negativity wastes time and energy that could be harnessed toward achieving your goals.

If you hone your positive thinking skills and develop the mental attitudes of a winner, you'll be able to overcome challenges without giving up. No matter how discouraging things may get or how intently others may try to dissuade you, with your winning attitude, you will be unstoppable!

A positive outlook enables you to focus on your goals with a tunnel vision that eliminates negative distractions and keeps you on a chartered course to success. We need to train our minds to focus on the good.

We often worry about our body shape but we should more often be concerned about the state of our thinking. Just as we train our bodies for peak performance, we must also train our minds by coaching ourselves to think winning thoughts. An effective way to train your mind is to look at challenges as opportunities instead of obstacles. A problem is only a problem if you allow it to be one. With each challenge comes an opportunity to learn and improve. So if you search for solutions, you'll find them.

5 Keys to a Healthy Mind

1. **Choose faith thoughts over fearful thoughts.**
   For God has not given us a spirit of fear, but of power and of love and of a sound mind.
   2 Timothy 1:7

2. **Chose stable thoughts over runaway emotions.**
   A sound mind makes for a robust body,
   but runaway emotions corrode the bones.
   Proverbs 14:30

3. **Choose peaceful thoughts over turmoil.**
   Don't sin by letting anger control you.
   Think about it overnight and remain silent.
   Psalm 4:4

4. **Choose God's Word over all other advice!**
   Oh, how I love your instructions!
   I think about them all day long.
   Psalm 119:97

5. **Choose to think before you act.**
   Wise people think before they act;
   fools don't—and even brag about their foolishness.
   Proverbs 13:16

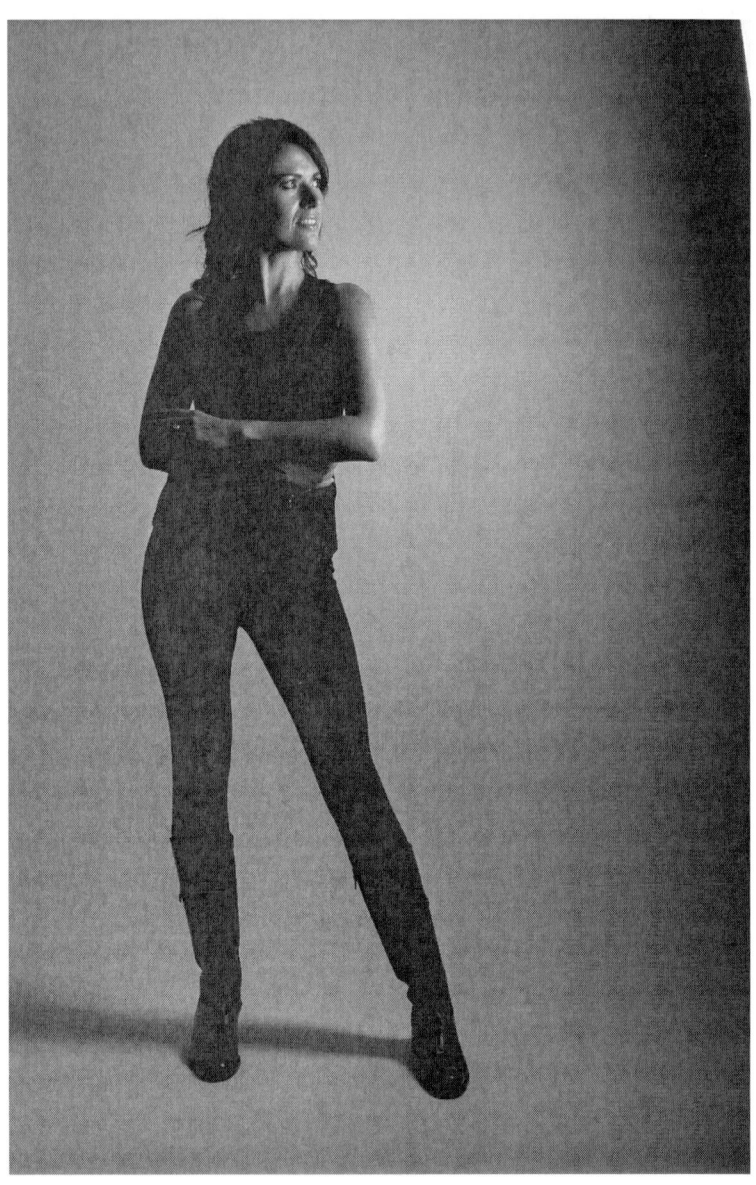

A strong mind makes for a strong body.

Chapter

20

Shape
That Body

To give definite form, shape, character to; fashion or form.

Exercise is something you simply cannot avoid if you want to fully achieve your body shaping dreams. I can say it fast if it helps, or even whisper it, but you cannot ignore it. You need to exercise. It's a no-go zone for some and a life-saving love for others. Although sitting is better than lying down, and standing is better than sitting, walking is much better than standing, but running is not better than walking [unless, of course, you're really fit]. Confused? Read on.

Let's explore the reasons why anyone should bother with exercise if they are getting good results from the Body

& Soul Lifestyle without moving a muscle [which will happen].

Your body's ability to burn fat is very much dependent on the tone of your muscles. If they are strong and well-toned, you will be a far more efficient fat-munching machine. Now, I don't know about you, but if doing a little exercise will make the whole body shaping thing a little easier, I for one am going to do it. By taking part in some focused exercise, you can consume more foods that you enjoy, and at the same time turn even your everyday movements into efficient, fat-burning activities [mini workouts without you even realizing that you're exercising].

> How you feel plays a large part in how you look.

Already, by following the Body & Soul Lifestyle, you will notice that you are sleeping better, and that you have more energy. This is great, but there's more! I'm sure you'll agree, if something makes you feel and perform better than you were previously, it's going to be a pleasure to continue it and make it a routine part of your life. Exercise releases hormones called endorphins which are responsible for your body's feeling of well-being. If done correctly, the right type of exercise will help your body to increase its ability to produce these natural feel-good hormones, and therefore also increase your ability to cope with stress, worry, or just twenty-first century living!

Although the Body & Soul Lifestyle is primarily a way of life that will ensure you have a better body shape, it also has another very positive side-effect – great health! Unfortunately, most methods used to change body shapes have detrimental effects on the body's health, especially in the long-term. This lifestyle does just the opposite. And, if you include some body shaping exercise in your new lifestyle, you are increasing the value of the body shaping 'insurance policy' you have just taken out by reading this book. It is literally a deposit, in your favor, in the body shaping bank! Regular muscular stimulation is the only way, combined with good nutrition, to ensure maximum health, mobility and youthfulness as you age.

> "Use it or lose it."
> One of the most important clichés ever quoted.
> Ignore it at your own risk.

So, what does it take? First of all, it's vital that you understand what exercise is before you can take part in it properly. You may have had quite extensive contact with various types of gym exercise, such as aerobics, pump, jump, thump, step, spin, Tai-Bo and circuit classes, or sports such as running, swimming, tennis or basketball. You probably undertook this type of exercise with many good intentions, but more often than not, without the results which were promised or expected. You may think it's your own fault for not being diligent enough, but it's usually true that it's just that you weren't doing the correct type of exercise to benefit a great body shape.

> Doing 50% of the right kind of exercise is far better than doing 100% of the wrong kind.

If you enjoy playing tennis, racquetball, volleyball or basketball, by all means, keep playing. But if you think it's all you need to get in shape, think again. Body shaping is definitely not a hit-and-miss thing. You can't just dip your hand into a big bag of activities and hope to achieve your goals by your good intentions, and a bit of sweat and luck to boot! If you consider body shaping a sport, then it may be easier to understand. Just as great swimmers don't play basketball to win the Olympic Games, and tennis players don't surf to win the US Open, it's important for you to understand that to achieve a better body shape, you have to train like a body shaper.

Have you ever seen an out of shape aerobics instructor or personal trainer? Every gym has at least one. Now why is it that these instructors, who take far more high-energy classes than you each week, are still overweight? Because they're usually eating wrong – overloading on carbs – to the extent that even the several cardio classes each week can't shift the fat. Can you see the equation here? High-impact cardio classes just do not equal fat loss and better body shape.

And it's not just cardio classes that shake the equation. Add to it running, jogging, circuit classes and any other high-energy activity. Why? Fat is a slow-burning energy. It is converted very slowly for use as a steady, long-lasting energy source.

> Fat must have oxygen to allow it to burn in the same way as a flame needs oxygen.

High-energy, high-impact activities demand a fast supply of fuel to keep them going. They also need a fuel that doesn't rely on oxygen: chances are you will be out of breath [in oxygen debt], so at these times the body will choose one of its fast energy providers, such as carbohydrates or glycogen energy. Therefore, little or no fat is burned by doing these types of activities.

"Oh, no!", I hear you groan. Wasted years jumping around for nothing. Well, not entirely. Your fitness level will have improved and you will have toned certain muscles to some degree. You will also have stimulated your metabolism to work a little faster, but as I mentioned earlier, you should now be only interested in the 100% optimum most efficient ways to get in shape, so please, don't knock yourself out wasting any more time!

Chapter

21

Start Today

This present time; now.

Have you ever wondered why exercise is so hard? If your answer is 'yes', you are not alone. I spent years pondering this same question, and in my endeavors to find a shortcut to the whole cardio and gym scenario, I discovered the answer to the dilemma. Training my mind. The main reason exercise is hard and not easy for many people is because they don't know how the body works and exactly what is needed to obtain a healthy and toned body shape.

For me, being 75 pounds overweight meant that there was a strain on my body and my soul. It was so difficult for me to exercise because of carrying around so much excess weight. My joints ached and everything was such an effort.

I started with walking and then after I had dropped the first 25 pounds I started with weights. And I haven't looked back. 75 pounds later exercise has become easier and easier and more and more enjoyable. Why? Because I am in better shape now and there is less of me to move!

But there was no getting around the fact that I had to start somewhere at some point in time and I knew that the hardest time would be the beginning. And in the beginning you require determination more than just about anything else.

> It is positively, absolutely, completely possible for you to be toned where you'd never dreamed it would be possible.

I love and believe in people, and I am aware of the pain that people go through with regards to how they feel and look. I want to see you set completely free.

It doesn't matter what age you are, or what stage you're at physically. You should be – we all should be – ready to become more active. And there is no better time than right now to say YES, instead of the usual, 'I'm starting back at the gym on Monday' routine! [You no doubt know what I mean!] Why not start on a Tuesday! Monday is the most tried and failed day of the week to start a new exercise plan.

Although most people can afford to become much more active, there is a small group of people who fall into the exceptional 'over-exercising' category; they enjoy doing torturously difficult exercise just for the sake of it. If that's you, my advice would be slow down, and take a good look at why you do what you do!

> Starting on a Monday holds about as much promise as your last New Year's Resolution!

It's my aim to turn the technical difficulties into body shaping simplicities. Unless you are an elite athlete or professional sports person, you really should be able to take part in some body shaping exercise, with great results.

Making time for exercise is important. Sometimes being busy is deceiving, and not necessarily constructive. We can be so busy with things that eat away at our time, without even being fully aware of them. Especially when you have a family.

> Something has to give way somewhere, and it's usually our health.

Looking after yourself may be a sacrifice. If you don't have time to exercise, then you have to choose to create some time, by giving your well-being some priority over other things or tasks.

For some people, it's a matter of life or death! It's pointless to be concerned about making money and spending more time with your family if you are going to kill yourself with a heart attack because of a poor diet and lack of exercise. Let's be realistic about what's REALLY important and what's not. You have to be around to enjoy your family and spend your money. So let's do something about that!

To ensure that you walk for 45-60 minutes, 4-5 days a week, you may have to wake up an hour earlier.

> One of the requirements of a leader is energy.
> J. Oswald Sanders

Statistics show that 75% of people who say they will exercise in the morning actually do, and only 25% of people who say they will exercise in the evening actually do. This is enough reason to aim for the morning. If something has to go at the end of a busy day, it's usually exercise. Bring it to the beginning of your day, and watch it change your life – for the better.

> Sow sparingly and you will reap sparingly.
> Sow abundantly and you will reap abundantly.
> 1 Corinthians 9:6

If we are going to live a high-energy lifestyle, then we have to sow high-energy. The answer to having more energy is not having more sleep or even having more rest. A recent survey found that 95% of people in the western world look forward to their weekends, but 52% of them feel more tired after their weekend than before. If we want to maximize our potential in life, we need to live a high-energy lifestyle.

Have you ever thought that you'd like to feel less tired and be able to achieve more? If you want a high-energy life, you need to sow energy to reap it. The more you expend energy, the more energy you will have. Guaranteed! The more energy you try to conserve, the less energy you will have. Guaranteed! Remember, you reap what you sow.

> Regular exercise = abundant energy.
> No exercise = next to no energy.
> You choose!

When you exercise, don't think about how much energy you are expending – instead think about how much energy you will reap as a result of the energy you sow. It's worth it!

Chapter

22

Fat Burning Cardio

To use fat as fuel.

Walking is probably the best fat-burning method known. It's also the easiest and least likely to cause injury, so use it. Cycling is also good. The trick is to keep to a good pace for as long as possible, without being completely breathless. This will guarantee you are burning fat. Wearing a heart rate monitor and having it set correctly will help you determine the best pace for you to be burning fat.

What's best about fat burning is that it can be done almost any time, anywhere, from a walk to and from work, or parking the car a little further from the office, or pushing your baby around the park. So do try and find thirty minutes or more each day, to make a big difference to your results.

> A brisk dawn or dusk walk clears away the cobwebs and helps you think.

With fat burning taken care of, let's now deal with another issue. I'm not going to give you a list of regular bum, tum and thigh exercises. They are probably why you've bought this book – because they haven t worked for you! It's not just the exercise you do, but it is, more importantly, how you do them.

I have absolutely no objection to any sport or current exercise program you may already enjoy. Keep it up if it's having the desired effect, that is, if it's increasing your fitness level, if your social or competitive needs are met, and if it is important to you. Basically, do it for pleasure, if you wish.

The more fat burning cardio and weights you do, the more weight you can expect to lose in the shortest amount of time possible. A woman can expect to lose 2.5 pounds per week and a man can expect to lose up to 5 pounds per week. Some things in life are just not fair!

Walking is definitely my number one choice for those who want to lose weight, and you don't need training to learn how to do it!

Over the years I have walked with my Dad, my sister Kathy, my friends, and these days I really love to go for 'walk and talk' time with my husband Jonathan.

WHEN TO WALK?

Mornings are the best time of day to do your cardio, to ensure that you are able to fit everything else into a busy schedule. There are also very good metabolic reasons for walking first thing in the morning. It actually gives your metabolism a kick-start for the day, which means fat burning! Winter is a little more difficult as all is dark outside early in the morning – but just think, you'll be home in time to see the sun rise!

If you have decided to exercise each day, by doing it in the morning you are not only making it a priority, but you are basically getting it out of the way so you can focus on everything else. Otherwise, if you decide to walk in the evening, but run out of time, you will go to bed feeling like a failure, and that's extra pressure you do not need.

It would be good for you to walk in the morning, if you can. If not, it would be good for you to walk … full stop!

WHERE TO WALK?

I choose to walk around where I live which is around a 4 mile circuit, which includes a couple of good inclines. It doesn't matter really where you choose to walk, but remember to keep the scenery as varied as possible, so you don't become bored.

Safety is also an issue. If you walk alone, it's important to take care, and it would be better for you not to walk alone in the evening. I know where I walk, there are many people out and about 'doing their thing' at 6am, so it's a good safe place to be, and, of course, I have someone to walk with, too!

There are other alternatives, such as walking in a low impact cardio class. Just be sure that your heart rate remains consistent and that you are moving for at least 45 minutes. This is the best fat burning time.

Another alternative is walking the treadmill at the gym, or using an elliptical which is better for your joints. A step machine is also excellent, and a great workout for your legs and backside.

The main thing is that you are able to walk somehow, some way. Walk where you won't be distracted, and walk where you have some good hills to help increase your fitness levels.

WHAT PACE AND FOR HOW LONG?

There's walking and there's WALKING. When I talk about walking, be assured, I'm talking about WALKING! This is at a considerable pace. Shoulders back, head up, walking at around 135 beats per minute. You should be able to hold a light conversation, but not be able to sing!

When you're walking, you should be breathing primarily through your nose and not your mouth, i.e. breathe normally! And, although you are feeling puffed, be assured that in a week or so your fitness levels will increase and increase. Basically you can only get fitter! Although walking three times a week for 20 minutes is better than not walking at all, it's really only a warm-up, and not very good for fat burning and muscle toning, which is really why you're doing it! The best length of time to walk is for 45-60 minutes, and the best number of days to walk each week is 4-6. Anything under that is okay, but your results will be in proportion with the amount of time and effort you put in.

WHAT ABOUT FOOD AND DRINKS?

It's so important that you remember to take at least 30oz of water with you when you are doing any form of physical exercise, including and especially walking. You may not think you will need it when you first step out, but you'll certainly be glad you brought it along at the end of a 4 mile walk! The main thing to remember in combining your food with your exercise is: don't eat before you exercise. The only people I know who eat before they exercise are certain male and female athletes who require a carbohydrate boost. Most of us, however, don't need a carbohydrate boost! Our biggest problem, besides eating too much fat, is an overload of carbohydrates.

The best thing to do is have plenty of water, day and night and especially when you're exercising. You may eat your breakfast as soon as you come home from your walk, if you are able to walk first thing in the morning. This will also help to keep your metabolic rate at a speedy pace throughout the day. Stay away from sports drinks unless you are being coached to drink them for training purposes. They are usually loaded with sugar. For you, good old-fashioned water should suffice.

WHAT DO I WEAR?

Something you may notice when you begin walking, especially after the first few days, is that you will need some good walking shoes. Your shins and ankles will soon let you know by aching day and night until you do something about it. What you need to look for in a suitable walking shoe is a good heel cushion, a flexible forefoot, plenty of room in the 'toe box' so that the shoes can spread during push-off, supporting heel construction for stability, and a low heel. Most sporting goods stores today have trained consultants on hand who are skilled at knowing which shoes will be best for the type of training you will be doing, coupled with the type of feet you have.

Make sure that you're dressed comfortably and coolly when you're exercising. Simple shorts or track pants with a t-shirt, and don't forget good supportive underwear – it's a must! It's also an idea to wear a hat, sunscreen and sunglasses if you decide to walk after around 7.30am in summer and 8.30am in winter.

The issue of hand weights has been debated by medical and exercise professionals for years. If you have high blood pressure, it's best that you walk without them. If, however, you are healthy, you can walk with them. Make sure you use your arm and shoulder muscles. Don't leave the weights dangling from your fingertips, and make sure you don't grip them too tightly.

WHY DO I STILL FEEL LIKE RUNNING?

Who knows! Except, many people do! I can understand if you still feel like running, even though I have told you to start walking, especially if you have always run and you are fairly active. But, I do need to stress that you consider why it is that you are running. If you want to run or jog for fitness – heart and lung fitness – go for it! If it's to get into shape, then slow down! Unless you are already fit, all you will be doing by running or jogging is working at a rate which doesn't allow the body to absorb oxygen properly, so it uses other energies, because fat needs oxygen to burn!

If you want to burn fat, walk until you become fitter, then if you really like jogging or running, then slowly, slowly, slowly pick up the pace until you are not breathless. Running on pavement may cause long-term joint injuries, so be sure to use a treadmill, if you can. Remember, it's more important to not be breathless than it is for you to run a single mile! It really is re-education. You may need to re-train your mind, and try it out for yourself. Go for it!

12 Ways to Burn [at least] 100 Calories

1. Pedal an exercise bike for 15 minutes.

2. Hike up hill for 15 minutes.

3. Clean the garage for 15 minutes.

4. Dance for 15 minutes.

5. Work in the garden for 30 minutes.

6. Swim for 20 minutes.

7. Mowing the lawn for 20 minutes.

8. Walk briskly for 20 minutes.

9. Clean the house for 25 minutes.

10. Play golf [with a cart] for 30 minutes.

11. Walking the dog [leisurely] for 45 minutes.

12. Putting away the groceries and light housework for 40 minutes.

Chapter

23

Muscle Toning and Strengthening

To gain strength; grow stronger.

I can remember nearly knocking myself out session after session, trying to cram in up to ten cardio classes a week, which was supposed to help me achieve all over muscle tone. Then I discovered resistance training, and everything changed from then on. Using weights, or resistance training, offers tremendous body shaping benefits. Resistance training is any exercise that involves the muscles of the body attempting to move some type of opposing force. As a muscle is used, it is strengthened and toned. The more it's used, the more strengthened and toned it will be.

As you lift a window that may be a little stiff, you can feel the resistance in your forearms, biceps and the front of your shoulders. Just as the window force is downwards, and you are lifting upwards, there you have a form of resistance exercise.

It's important to remember when you are doing resistance training that you actually feel resistance in your muscles. If you don't feel that they are being 'worked', then they probably are not being 'worked'. On the other hand, it's important for you to get to know your body, and to get a feel for what muscle resistance is, and the feeling of using your muscles, versus pain in the joints, tendons and ligaments. It's good to 'feel' what your muscles are doing. It should feel 'hard', but not feel overly 'painful'. If any exercise feels too painful, you should stop immediately, and seek professional advice from a registered fitness expert.

I have the most amazing Personal Trainer and for me, it is all about the extra 10% I can't achieve by myself. Michelle is incredible – the best I have ever known, and she always pushes me beyond me and shows me what's really in me... That is a value to my life, at my age and stage, that I can't put a price on!

We all want to feel great and look great, and be free to live the life we were created to live. In many studies carried out by various health and fitness organizations, it has been found that muscle training helps to keep us young. Now that's something we ALL want to know about! This relates to an increase in fitness, a decline in stress levels, an increase in muscular tone strength, a stability of bone density and good joint flexibility. All things we would certainly notice if we were without them!

The truth is, you do not need to do a lot of different exercises, only a few very basic ones, done correctly, to take you a long way towards your body toning goals.

Again, I want to encourage you to weigh up the initial 'discomfort' of exercise against years of being unhappy with yourself. You can plod away for years and years, watching cardio videos and taking part as much as you can, and you won't see a fraction of the improvement that you will once you begin walking and using resistance training to tone your muscles.

Once you decide to get serious about what you really want, you are going to see for yourself how easy it all is – really!

> Weights or resistance training is the quickest proven method to change your body shape with the minimum amount of effort.

If you already consider yourself a 'fitness fanatic', then you will be aware of the incredible benefits of training with weights. If however, you are the exact opposite, then I'm here to help you become aware of the benefits!

Cardio exercise, such as walking, is great for improving cardiovascular fitness [your heart], and improving muscular endurance in your legs, but contributes only a small amount to toning the rest of your body, and improving your overall flexibility, muscular endurance and strength, especially in your upper body.

Weight training is an activity that can be done in a short period, yet it makes dramatic changes to your body shape – and how you feel. Having toned muscles not only feels great, it also increases your energy level and improves your productivity at work and in many other everyday activities.

Training with weights helps to maintain muscle strength, muscular endurance, nerve-muscle [neuromuscular] co-ordination, and bone density, which helps to prevent osteoporosis, not to mention a whole range of other nasty medical conditions.

Research shows us that weight training makes a significant contribution to quality of life, whatever one's age or gender. And remember, it is a fat burning exercise!

One of the most difficult thought processes I had to overcome at first was that if I did any exercise with weights, that would mean that I would grow massive muscles, and end up looking like the Incredible Hulkess! However, this was not so! I discovered that to grow huge muscles took huge effort, huge amounts of body-building foods, and often, huge amounts of steroids. So relax and know that your muscles are only going to become as big and toned as they can naturally, which can be very attractive.

> Weight training is for *everybody*,
> not just a select few.

If you know all your hard work is going to hit the mark, you'll invest much more time and energy into doing it. One of the greatest hurdles I had to overcome was moving from training in the aerobics room to training in the weights room – with all the big and sweaty 'grunters'. Many years ago, training with weights was not heard of for any other purpose than bodybuilding, weight lifting, or for other sports which required great power and strength. The weight room was hardly the place to find a novice who simply wanted to get into better shape! How times have changed! We now recognize that weight training was the best way all along.

I discovered that I was able to broaden my shoulder width by doing certain shoulder exercises and was able to tone up the back of my legs and buttocks by doing various hamstring and glute [bottom] exercises.

You may already be aware of all the wonderful benefits of resistance training. If not, I want to encourage you not to feel intimidated by something new, and something which has before now been associated with unwarranted fears about growing BIG unsightly muscles! It takes a lot of time, energy, food [and steroids] to become a bulky looking body builder. It can't and won't happen accidentally, so have no fear!

It wasn't until I started resistance training that I finally had the true results I wanted. Doing cardio was keeping me fit on the inside, which is important, but the muscle tone just wasn't there. When I started to use weights, the shape of my legs changed, and I became much stronger and fitter in the process.

Instead of having string-bean legs, I actually developed some shape in the front of my thighs. And, even more amazingly, my inner thighs and back of my thighs slimmed right down and toned right up, in proportion with the rest of my legs.

Until I properly understood the body shaping benefits of resistance training, I limited myself to simply dreaming about any kind of substantial improvement.

One great result of resistance training is that it will help give you the ability to go shopping and carry massive loads of shopping bags without any difficulty! Your back will be strengthened and your shoulders and arms will be much stronger than ever before. And you won't bulge with massive muscles, but instead you will have nicely toned muscle shape.

Another great result of resistance training is that your stamina is increased. You will no longer be lethargic and out of breath when walking or climbing stairs, but instead feel as though a huge weight has been lifted from your shoulders. It's time to lean against the right wall, to walk up the right path, to do those things that will take us to the right place faster! If you are doing countless amounts of exercise already and not getting the results you need, it's time to stop and re-evaluate how you are spending your time.

> If the ladder is not leaning against the right wall, every step you take just gets you to the wrong place faster!
> Stephen R. Covey

First of all you need to ensure that you are feeding your muscles properly with a good diet, high in protein. You also need to ensure that the exercise you are doing is helping your body to become the fat burning, muscle toning, energy building machine that it was created to be.

HOW LONG AND HOW HARD SHOULD I TRAIN?

Although there is an obvious advantage with walking, as you don't require equipment, there is an even greater advantage in your body toning progress with weight training. Unlike other exercise activities that rely on developing specific muscles, for example, legs for walking or cycling, weight training programs can be designed to develop your legs as well as many other muscle groups.

You would be surprised with the fitness levels of many body-builders who don't run marathons, but instead walk, cycle or use a stepper machine, and train with weights. Those who train consistently are extremely fit! Training with weights can be a 'cardio', fat burning experience when done properly. Providing the training session is approximately 45 minutes in length, and is carried out at a heart rate of approximately 135 beats per minute, then your fitness level will rise, and fat burning will take place.

The way I train is without rest in between sets. I also train differently every session – making sure that my muscles don't know what's going on.

Initially I was training with weights 4 days per week, but I only did this for 12 weeks. After the 12 weeks, I have been training 2 days per week, which is optimum for rest and muscle strengthening and toning.

By increasing muscle tone [and they don't have to be huge], you are making your body into a well-tuned machine, able to burn fat. If your body has well-toned muscle tissue, and you eat a well-balanced diet with plenty of protein and water, it will always use up its store of fat first!

This means that once you have improved your muscle tone through weight training, and you have been eating right, you are able to be less strict with your food intake.

It's a fact that the difference between people who are overweight and those who are not is not necessarily the food intake as much as the lack of physical activity.

If you can't exercise for whatever reason, you are still able to have a great body shape through eating right, but if you want a great body shape which is toned and which frees you up from being so strict with your food intake, then walk and train with weights. It's that simple!

What makes weight training exciting is the rapid rate at which you can see and feel changes in your body! As soon as you begin exercising, your muscles feel firmer, and the body toning process begins. Regular training will convince you that you have the ability to tone your body better than you may ever have expected!

Although you can't grow new muscles, you can change the tone and shape of your muscles, whatever your body type, and so bridge the gap between the physique you want and the one you look at every day in the mirror! Toned muscles look and feel great; they don't droop at the back of your arms, or sag at your waist. If you follow the instructions properly in this book, you will find this out for yourself!

HOW OFTEN SHOULD I TRAIN?

You should exercise two to three times each week to achieve good muscle tone. Weight training more than that really won't speed your progress, as recovery time in between training sessions is very, very important. Sometimes, the greatest enthusiasts end up being the most injured! Once you've made up your mind to train with weights, it's important to take it one step at a time, and if you're a beginner, then start as a beginner. It's pointless knocking yourself out in the first week, and then being

205 Body & Soul by Dianne Wilson

unable to train for the next three weeks because you're too sore and can't move!

The length of your training session will depend on what stage you're up to and which body parts you're training. Somewhere between 30 and 45 minutes is a good indication. You should be training hard. This doesn't mean that you should be trying to kill yourself, but you should be using effort in everything you do. Just as when you're walking it's important to walk with good posture and to concentrate on the muscles you're using, the same applies to weight training. If you can concentrate on what you're doing, you will tone your muscles in a much shorter period of time. If you squeeze your legs while doing lunges, for example, your legs will be getting a double workout, in half the time, and the benefits are twice as impressive! And when you're doing lunges, make sure your knees are over your toes and only do lunges backwards rather than forwards. This will give you a fantastic workout and will help ensure you don't injure your knees.

WHERE SHOULD I TRAIN?

The obvious and best place to train, if you can afford it, is your local gym. They have spent literally hundreds of thousands of dollars on equipment and maintenance of equipment, for you to benefit from. All you have to do is turn up, use it at your leisure, and leave, without giving it a second thought – except, of course, for the initial gym membership cost.

If you decide to set up a home gym, you may like to first consider the cost, then the inconvenience of having equipment taking up space in your home. There is the advantage of privacy if you'd like it, but exercising can become boring if you don't have any contact with anyone.

The best solution, if you can't afford gym membership, is to buy yourself a good pair of dumbbells and use them at home. Sometimes it's not even money – it's time and convenience, as I've mentioned previously. If you have kids at home, or if you work odd hours, you are much better off following a routine that doesn't mean you have to be somewhere else to do it.

Put up pictures of what the new you is going to look like, and empty out your kitchen cupboards and fridge. If you're going to train at home, at least make it easier on yourself!

WHAT ABOUT MY AGE AND STAGE?

I don't believe there should be any limits placed on anyone because of age and stage of development. Probably the youngest suggested age for weight training is around 16 years, to be safe, although there are a number of teenagers, especially guys, who start earlier than this. Teenagers should be careful with weight training to ensure that their bones have developed sufficiently to cope with the weights being used.

As far as the other end of the scale is concerned, it doesn't matter how old you are either. The earlier you start and the more consistent you are with weights, the longer you will look and feel great. If you are a beginner, take heart – you won't be for long. Everybody has to start somewhere at some time, and if this is your time – great! Before too long you will be glad you decided to do something about your physique that would be long lasting in appearance, and fun in the process.

A lean, well-proportioned body *only* comes from losing body fat and gaining muscle!

CAN I 'SPOT REDUCE'?

One vital point to remember is that you cannot 'spot reduce'. In other words, if you have a roll of fat on your tummy, doing 1000 sit-ups three times a day is not going to get rid of it. The result of this type of over-exercising will widen the stomach, not slim it!

You will not necessarily be burning fat from the area you are training. The reason you are doing weight resistance training is to firm your muscles and increase your body's ability as a whole to burn fat from wherever it sees fit. And believe me, it's often not our choice of fat store that goes first, e.g. breasts or face. In fact, the general rule is, the bigger the fat store – e.g. bottom, hips and thighs – the more it is likely that the body will leave it until last. So it's vitally important to be patient, and persistent – especially now that you know why. The best part of living this lifestyle is that you will notice body fat gone from places you never thought possible! Don't give up!

GOOD POSTURE

One of the most important factors when doing any kind of physical exercise is posture. If you have good posture, you are already off to a good start. If not, it's the first thing I want to work on with you.

If your posture is not good, it needs correcting. If you don't correct your posture, and you begin exercising, especially with weights, all you will be doing is adding to your problem.

If your shoulders are already rounded because of the way you have stood or sat for years and years, it's now time to straighten up! If you don't, you may injure your joints and tendons.

So, shoulders back, head up, joints slightly relaxed to soften the stress, and off you go! Keep it simple – keep it possible and achievable!

SAFETY TIPS

Weight training includes the use of dumbbells, barbells, and/or machinery. When you are doing an exercise with a bar or dumbbells, it's important that you check that the weight is not too heavy for you. It's also important that you don't have it too light, as you won't improve unless your muscles are used!

If possible, exercise in front of a mirror, so you can continually check your form and posture.

If you are doing any exercise which requires you to lift the weight above your head, it would be wise for you to use a training partner to assist you, if necessary.

Always hold your stomach in tight while exercising. Not only does this provide good support for your lower back, but it will help tone your stomach muscles in the process!

During exercises where you are required to stand, always keep your knees slightly bent to ensure the muscles surrounding your knees are providing the necessary support.

If you are a beginner, lift light weights until you can perform a particular exercise correctly. Remember, good form is always more important than lifting heavy weights. If you have to hunch over, swing your back and break your arm to lift a mega-sized dumbbell, you are wasting your time.

When lifting heavy weights, always lift with your knees. Using the muscles in your hips and thighs, bend down to the weight and pick it up. Don't use your back – ever! This same rule applies when picking up anything heavy, be it groceries, children, anything!

It's important also to keep the weight close to your body. This will ensure controlled movement and beneficial muscle toning.

Remembering all the safety tips, you also need to know that to effectively train a muscle to become stronger and more toned, you need to stimulate your muscles by working them. This is called 'overload'. It means taking your muscles one step further in strength and endurance each time you use them.

You need to proceed carefully with overloading your muscles, as sometimes over-keenness can bring about injury. Gradually combine overload with rest, and remember that it's the overload which stimulates the muscles to be stronger and more toned, and it's the rest which provides the room to do so.

EQUIPMENT

Although many weight training exercises include the use of training equipment – dumbbells, barbells, or machinery – there should also be enough props around your home to keep you very busy in the comfort of your own home. Furniture, a broomstick and even a couple of cans of baked beans, instead of dumbbells, will work!

I do recommend, however, that you buy yourself a pair of dumbbells, as these aren't very expensive and will be most useful. Don't get them too light, but don't go overboard with weight if you are a beginner. If you're just starting out, somewhere between 5 pounds and 10 pounds for each dumbbell will be sufficient.

If you want to buy a bar without weights attached, these weigh around 15 pounds, which will give you good resistance. And, as you improve and become stronger, you can add weights to the ends of the bar.

An exercise mat is also a good idea for your floor exercises. If you don't have one, simply lay a towel down onto carpet. This is usually all the comfort you would get at the gym anyway!

There are many home gyms and machines available. The best thing to do is decide for yourself what you need them for and also consider the cost and space they take up.

If you can, find a good gym and buy yourself a membership, which will give easy access to all the equipment you will need. Shop around as some offer special deals to new clients.

> Remember your priorities!
> Train to look good, rather than worrying about looking good to train!

Always train in comfortable clothes and supportive shoes. If you are training at the gym, especially, wear something that can get dirty and sweaty. Please don't spend hundreds of dollars to make a fashion statement here – but spend it afterwards instead, by all means!

STRETCHING

It's important to prepare your body for exercise. Just as you prepare for work in the morning by having a shower, getting dressed and eating your breakfast, you need to prepare your body for exercise by warming up and stretching. If you don't prepare your muscles for exercise correctly, you will be prone to injuries, and that's the bottom line. You will get much more out of a muscle, the warmer it is. Once the blood is flowing to a particular muscle group, it is ready for exercise. You'll notice that professional dancers always warm up. You need to become a professional body toner. You always need to warm up. A good warm-up session can increase your metabolic rate, and hence, start fat burning before you even begin your training routine.

It's also important to cool down and stretch after exercising. I can remember numerous times when I've worked out with weights, and gone straight home in a rush before cooling down and stretching properly, only to find I couldn't move the next day, or three! Ouch!

UPPER BODY

> Broad shoulders, a taut chest, firm arms,
> toned stomach and strong back.
> You can do it!

Most people aren't aware of all the different muscles in their body. Biceps [front of upper arms], triceps [back of upper arm] and pectorals [chest] are probably the most well-known in the upper body. Together with trapezius [top of shoulders], deltoids [back of shoulders] and latissimus of the back [sides of the back], they make up the muscles associated with a classic physique.

The upper body has been shown through studies to suffer the most neglect. Without a strong upper half, it is impossible to even do one push-up! Women are renowned for being weak in the upper body, with flabbiness being a common problem in the back of their arms.

But the good news is that because the upper body is usually neglected, it is often quick to respond to training, and the results can be very impressive.

Broadened shoulders give an appearance that your hips are slimmer. Firmly toned arms look great in sleeveless tops and a strong back always looks great in a swimsuit or backless dress.

Because everyone is different with regards to strength and personal goals, it's important to determine what is going to be right for you. Make sure you don't become carried away with improving one body part, as this will lead to imbalance and can cause injury and joint problems.

It's really important, as I mentioned previously with regards to posture, that your body position is maintained during exercise. If you rock back and forth from the hips while doing bicep curls, for example, not only will this be easier for you, and therefore less effective, but you may even suffer back strain in the process. It's not worth cheating to make things easier, because in the long run, you won't achieve your goals, and you may land yourself a nasty injury.

Having a toned upper half means that your head is held erect, your chest is strong and uplifted, and your shoulders are relaxed and even. Opening heavy doors and carrying a dozen grocery bags should no longer pose a problem!

LOWER BODY

Your largest muscles, and potentially the most developed ones, are most likely to be found in your lower body. This is because your hips and legs have to support and move the rest of your body. For the average sized adult, this means carrying more than 100 pounds.

Your lower body muscles can be slower to show the effects of training, because of lack of use. In turn this lack of use can result in a more noticeable, saggy appearance.

Also, it can be harder to train and improve the lower body muscles because they aren't as easy to 'overload' as the upper body muscles.

However, all can be improved!

Muscle-toning exercises alone will not slim your thighs, but they will improve your appearance by firming and toning muscle tissue as you lose weight. The only way to lose fat and get rid of lumps and bumps is to watch what you're eating and increase your energy output.

A strong and well-toned lower half will make you feel great and look great. You will find that the more exercise you do with your lower body, the easier it will get. Remember though, careful overload is what brings about great results, so don't get lazy or too comfortable doing any exercises – especially with your legs and bottom!

If you've ever looked at some legs and wondered how it is that they have such great shape, it's either because of genetics, and good use of them [a mesomorph who uses what they have], or it's sheer hard work using resistance training [weights].

The great news is, because of resistance training, it doesn't matter what your current physical shape is - you can change it. Using weights is a body sculpting process where your muscle begins to strengthen and take great shape, and your body fat reduces through walking and eating healthily.

If you do 1000 sit-ups a day and don't change your eating habits, you won't change your stomach. But, if you eat healthily and do a sensible, well-balanced amount of exercise, your stomach will look outstanding, and in hardly any time at all!

Remember that balance is important. Not only balancing weights – so you don't drop them on your toes – but balancing the whole diet and exercise thing.

This is the bottom line – if you want to look great, feel great, work, sleep and play well, then you have to …

...eat well and exercise consistently
FOREVER!

Chapter

24

Zero In

To focus one's aim; to zoom in and center on something.

Most people know about lunges, leg raises and squats – the stuff that fitness videos get you doing in your living room. Exercise is a mind-blowing, complex issue, with numerous different types, styles and fads, and it's changing all the time. This is not a bad thing, as everybody has different responses to different types of exercise.

Even the old exercise DVD in your living room can work wonders when you know what you're doing and why. No matter how average the program you choose, or how little you know about training, if you follow exactly the following rules, it will work.

Focus is everything.

7 Keys to a Zeroing In

1. Find out exactly which area of your body you are working when you exercise. If you are not completely sure, ask someone who knows. It's the most crucial part of training. When you know it, write it down.

2. When doing the exercise, concentrate completely on the area you are supposed to be working. Don't think about what's for dinner, or where you have to be next, or what the kids are doing. We all know someone who has been training for years and still looks little different from when they started. Almost always this is due to lack of focus. They go through the motions without any thought to what is and isn't working. Don't waste your time – CONCENTRATE!

3. If you cannot feel an exercise in the area where you are supposed to, yet you are feeling it in an area you're not trying to work, simply adjust your position until you feel it where you should. Don't be afraid to shuffle your body into the correct position. Just because someone tells you that you are supposed to do it like this or that, it's irrelevant if you can't feel it, or if it's working a totally different area. Everyone is built differently, so make the exercise work for you.

4. Effort is vital. Do not worry about how many times you are supposed to repeat an exercise. The rule is easy – keep going until you can't go any more [at the same time, feeling it where you are supposed to], then stop

and rest until you feel ready. Then do it again. Repeat this three or four times, or even up to five times, depending on how you feel. Remember to monitor yourself carefully, so you don't overdo it in the beginning. Obviously, if you are unfit, you won't be able to do much, and if you are fit, you'll be able to do a lot more. By following this guideline, you will improve the muscle every time you train it, instead of stopping just about when the exercise starts to work for you.

5. Each time you do each exercise, push just a little more, building up slowly. It's a lot of fun and very inspirational to see how quickly you can improve.

6. Don't rush an exercise. Do them all slowly and deliberately, being aware of what is working through the up [bending or flexing] and the down [stretching or extending] of the movement.

7. Rest. Your body will not respond well if you don't allow it adequate time to rest. Always do weight training on alternate days rather than every day as your body needs rest time in between to rebuild.

In summary, by applying the above principles, you will guarantee results. It is essential, however, that you apply all of them all the time. They are quite literally the key that makes the difference between those who shape up and those who don't.

The following guide has been designed as a simple guide with which you can assess your own program. Do whatever you can fit into your schedule, and try to make improvements over time, as you become more comfortable with the exercise.

Body Shaping Exercise

TYPE OF EXERCISE	NO. OF DAYS PER WEEK	DURATION PER DAY
FAT BURNING Fast Walking	4-6 days	45-60 mins
MUSCLE TONING Weights	2-3 days	45-60 mins

Don't eat right before exercising, and try to eat 30 minutes after you've finished.

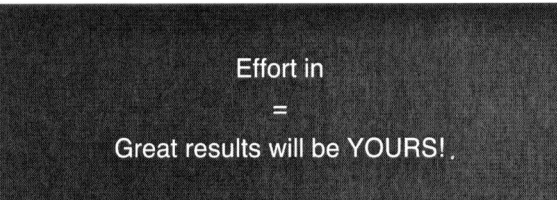

Effort in
=
Great results will be YOURS! .

Chapter

25

Exercise FAQ

An expression of inquiry that invites or calls for a reply.

WHEN WILL I SEE RESULTS?

You will start to actually feel different in two to three weeks, and begin to look different in three to five weeks. The most dramatic results will come in six to eight weeks. This is when it will show not only in your physique, but also in your face. People will ask you, 'What's different?', just as they would if you've had a new haircut. You won't look drawn and tired. You will have a greater energy level, and because you'll be sleeping better [a positive side effect of the Body & Soul Lifestyle], you will literally be bright eyed and bushy tailed! The results will keep on keeping on, for as long as you want. You may decide to be really careful for up to twelve weeks, then relax a little for the next week or two, then go back on for another four to six weeks. It can be in as many stages as you want.

WHEN CAN I WEIGH MYSELF?

Weigh yourself at least twice a week. And remember when you weigh in that muscle weighs three times more than fat. If you want to get a true picture of how well you're really doing with your new Body & Soul Lifestyle, check your weight and also check by tape measure. You will be dropping inches as well as pounds.

WHAT ABOUT AEROBICS?

Let's take a brief look at the aerobic activity which goes on at your local gym or health club, and how beneficial it actually is [or isn't] with regards to fat loss and muscle tone. One of the hardest things to do, especially if you have kids, is to wake up at some unearthly hour, switch on the TV [feeling absolutely gorgeous – not!], and suddenly find yourself watching half a dozen unbelievable bodies taking part in a perfectly choreographed aerobics routine.

It's 6am, and they're smiling – but you're not! Take heart. The fact of the matter is that these guys don't just do aerobics classes to look like that. They walk or do other cardio activities, each day, and they train in the gym – yes, with weights! If you enjoy doing aerobics classes, whether high or low, step, slide, box, funk, circuit, bums, tums or all of the above, by all means continue, but do consider why you are doing them!

WHAT ABOUT SPORTS?

Sports are great, and I encourage young people to take part in some type of sport each week, especially in their developing years. People involved in sports are usually outgoing, positive and energetic – the type of people that others like being around. However, it's important for us not to confuse these benefits with body shaping benefits. Body shapers, too, are usually outgoing and energetic, and their physical shape is one of the major benefits of playing their type of sport!

Although I encourage people to take part in sports, especially in my own family [my kids love soccer, swimming, hockey], it's another ball park when it comes to fat loss and muscle toning. If you are into sports [playing them, and not just watching them], and it's for fun or fitness – great! But, if it's only for fat loss and muscle toning – forget it!

You can still play sports because you enjoy them, but remember what I said about specificity of exercise and how important it is to be specific with what exercise you do.

HOW DO I MAINTAIN MY NEW BODY SHAPE?

By maintaining the Body & Soul Lifestyle. It's important to remember that you can do as much or as little of what has been suggested as you choose – and you can do it for as long or as short as you wish. If you want to maintain your new improved body shape, all you have to remember are the principles that gave you the new shape. When you've achieved your goal, your metabolism will be naturally faster, and you can probably even afford to occasionally have a couple of Treat Days per week.

Because of the foundation you have laid in stripping body fat instead of muscle tissue and water, you will find that weight doesn't pour back on if you go off the rails for a short while. Just remember what you put into achieving your new body shape, and that should be reason enough to keep a close check on what you eat in future.

HOW CAN SOME PEOPLE BE THIN, YET STILL FAT?

Ever noticed how even the skinniest girl in short shorts can still have dimply, flabby legs? This is because the muscle tissue has been starved by poor nutrition and severe lack of exercise. That's why even some 'bigger' girls look great, because they are a healthy size, with low body fat. It's the naked you which really counts and shows how healthy you are. I'd much rather be a healthy size 4-6 with no cellulite, thank you!

HOW LONG WILL IT TAKE FOR MY METABOLISM TO CHANGE?

The average time it takes for a sluggish metabolism to speed up is six to eight weeks. Of course, your genetics, fitness levels, and how careful you are at living the Body & Soul Lifestyle will determine how long it takes you personally. The main thing to remember is that if you live the lifestyle, your metabolism will change. So, be encouraged, have patience, and just keep going until it does!

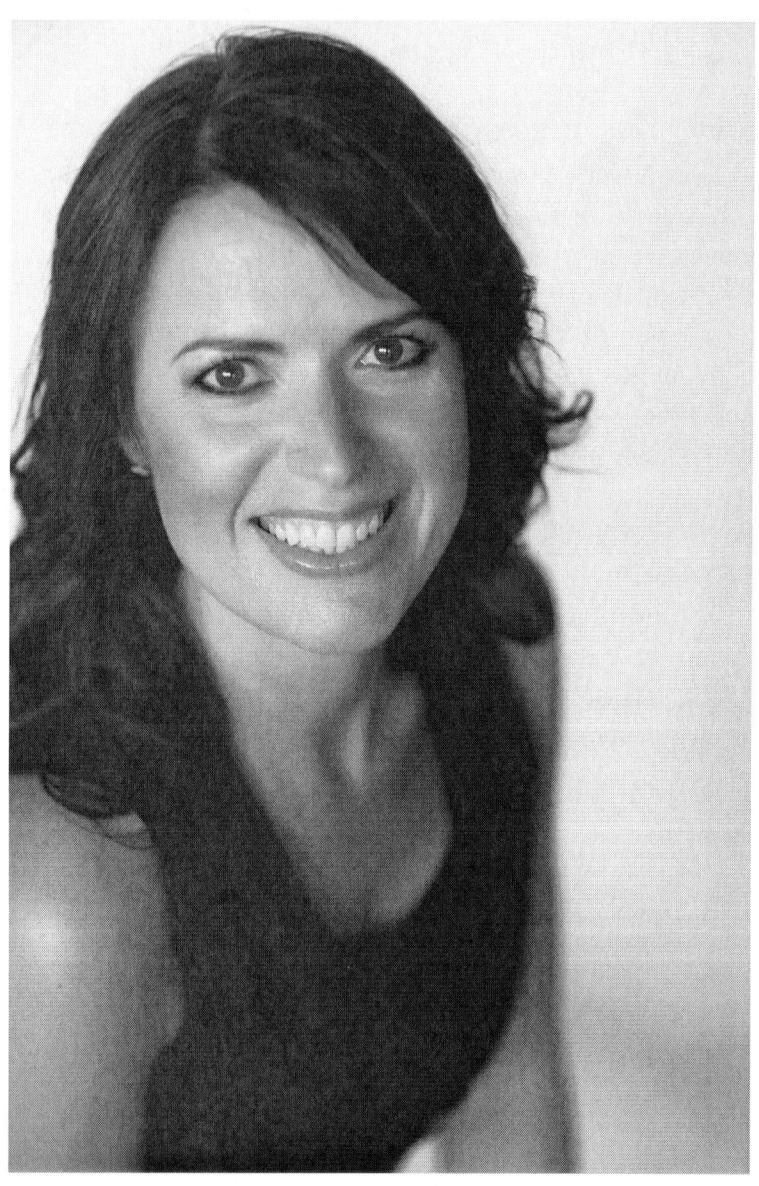

Let's cook!

body &soul

recipes

Body & Soul Recipes

What is unique about the Body & Soul Recipes is the coding guide, which has been designed to make life easier for you. You can quickly turn to any recipe and not have to work out what time of day it should be eaten. After a while you will become familiar with the recipes and will know when the best time to eat is for you. Remember, stay away from the pasta, potatoes and rice recipes until you have reached your goal weight. And then only eat very sparingly, but enjoy!

BODY & SOUL RECIPES CODING GUIDE
Each recipe has three faces at the top of the page.

B   **Breakfast**
L   **Lunch**
D   **Dinner**

☺   **eat it and enjoy**
[this is the best time of day to eat this meal]

☺   **eat it and enjoy eat it if you must**
[something else would be better]

☹   **don't eat it now!**
[choose something else as this isn't suitable now]

Contents

Contents *continued*

Contents *continued*

Contents *continued*

Body & Soul Favorites!

★   Farmhouse Muesli

★   Big Breakfast

★   Grilled Chicken with Tomatoes and Basil

★   Unfried Chicken Strips

★   Springtime Stir Fry

Farmhouse Muesli

B L D

20 minutes to make
Serves 2 adults

Ingredients
1/2 cup dried prunes
1/2 cup dried apricots
2 cups hot water
1 cup quick cooking oats
2 tablespoons low fat muesli
1 cup non-fat milk
1 cup water
2 servings protein powder [suitable for cooking]

Method
1. Heat prunes and apricots in hot water in the microwave for 10–20 minutes, depending on what type of microwave you have, and let sit until plump.
2. Into a medium non-stick saucepan, place oats, muesli, protein powder, water and milk. Stir thoroughly. If possible, allow to soak cold for 10–15 minutes.
3. Cook on a low to medium heat for approximately 10 minutes, ensuring a creamy texture. Add a little more milk if necessary. Make sure the mixture isn't gluggy.
4. Serve piping hot with warm prunes, apricots and honey, and a dollop of natural non-fat yogurt, if desired.

Big Breakfast

B L D

☺ 😐 ☹

20 minutes to make
Serves 2 adults

Ingredients

4 slices low fat smoked ham
1/2 cup fat free chicken stock
2 large ripe tomatoes
handful fresh button mushrooms
your choice of eggs

Method

1. Begin cooking ham in half the chicken stock in a small non-stick frying pan. Cover with a lid after one side has browned. Add a little extra water if necessary.
2. In a separate frying pan, cook the tomatoes in chunks, along with the mushrooms and the remaining chicken stock.
3. Cook your choice of eggs as per the recipes in the Eggs section.
4. Serve immediately with toast [no butter].

Grilled Chicken with Tomatoes and Basil

B L D

20 minutes to make
Serves at least 4 adults

Ingredients

4 chicken breasts washed and trimmed.
2 cans whole peeled tomatoes
2 teaspoons fresh or 1 teaspoon dried basil
½ teaspoon salt
½ teaspoon pepper
¼ cup chopped spring onions
1 teaspoon crushed garlic
¼ cup red wine

Method

1. Brush the chicken breasts with a little olive oil and season with salt and pepper.
2. Grill the chicken on a barbeque grill or inside grill.
3. Place the rest of the ingredients in a medium-sized non-stick saucepan. Stir well and simmer on low–medium heat for 30 minutes, or until liquid is fairly reduced.
4. Pour the sauce over the chicken.
5 Serve with a fresh green leafy salad

Unfried Chicken Strips

B L D

15 minutes to make
Serves 4 adults

Ingredients

3 double chicken breast fillets [skinless and boneless]
¾ cup Cajun spices
4 eggs [1 yolk only]
1/3 cup teriyaki sauce
pepper and salt to taste

Method

1. Wash chicken and remove any traces of fat. Cut each half breast into 4 strips.
2. Empty the spices, salt and pepper in a bowl with the eggs and teriyaki sauce and whisk well.
4. Heat a large non-stick frying pan on high until the pan is really hot.
5. Dip each chicken strip in the mixture then place strips straight into the hot pan and cover with a lid.
7. After 5–7 minutes, turn the strips over [they should look greyish]. Replace the lid and cook a further 3–4 minutes.
8. Remove lid and splash a little water over chicken so it starts to look golden. Replace lid. Turn and splash until the golden color comes through most of each strip.
9. Cook for a further 2 minutes. Remove.
   This frying/steaming combination creates a great taste while keeping the chicken moist and succulent.

Springtime Stir Fry

B L D

20 minutes to make
Serves 4 adults

Ingredients
2 cups fresh green beans
1 cup fresh snow peas
1 cup shredded cabbage
1/2 cup bean sprouts
1/2 cup fat free vegetable stock
1 teaspoon Cajun spices salt and pepper to taste
1/2 cup white wine

Method
1. Preheat a large non-stick frying pan while preparing vegetables.
2. Combine all the ingredients, place in frying pan and place a lid on top.
3. After 10 minutes or so, stir and replace the lid.
4. Remove when veggies are just cooked.
5. Serve hot on its own, or with some grilled chicken strips.

Protein Shakes

★   Berry Smoothie

★   Kiwi, Lime & Mint Shake

★   Apple Crush

★   Iced Coffee Shake

★   Chocolate Delight

Berry Smoothie

B L D

2 minutes to make
Serves 1 adult

Ingredients
1 serving of protein powder
1/2 cup fresh berries
1 tablespoon plain low fat yogurt
1 teaspoon honey
1 cup non-fat milk
1 cup water

Method
1. Using a container which will hold up to 3 cups of liquid, pour in the milk. [Make sure the milk is added first!]
2. Add the other ingredients.
3. Blend well.
4. Drink right away while chilled, or take with you in a container to drink throughout the day.

Kiwi, Lime & Mint Shake

B L D

2 minutes to make
Serves 1 adult

Ingredients
1 serving of protein powder
1 kiwi fruit
1 tablespoon plain low fat yogurt
1 teaspoon honey
1/2 a lime, juiced
sprig of fresh mint
1 cup non-fat milk
1 cup water

Method
1. Using a container which will hold up to 3 cups of liquid, pour in the milk. [Make sure the milk is added first!]
2. Add the other ingredients.
3. Blend well.
4. Drink right away while chilled, or take with you in a container to drink throughout the day.

Apple Crush

B L D
☺ ☺ ☺

2 minutes to make
Serves 1 adult

Ingredients
1 serving of protein powder
1 whole apple cored
1 tablespoon plain low fat yoghurt
1 cup non-fat milk
1 cup water
1 cup ice

Method
1. Using a container which will hold up to 3 cups of liquid, pour in the milk. [Make sure the milk is added first!]
2. Add the other ingredients.
3. Blend well.
4. Drink right away while chilled, or take with you in a container to drink throughout the day.

Iced Coffee Shake

B L D

  ☺

2 minutes to make
Serves 1 adult

Ingredients

1 serving of protein powder
½ cup fresh espresso coffee
1 teaspoon artificial sweetener
1 cup non-fat milk
1 cup water

Method

1. Using a container which will hold up to 3 cups of liquid, pour in the milk. [Make sure the milk is added first!]
2. Add the other ingredients.
3. Blend well.
4. Drink right away while chilled, or take with you in a container to drink throughout the day.

Chocolate Delight

B L D

2 minutes to make
Serves 1 adult

Ingredients

1 serving of protein powder
2 teaspoons low fat drinking chocolate powder or liquid
1 cup non-fat milk
1 cup water
1 cup ice

Method

1. Using a container which will hold up to 3 cups of liquid, pour in the milk. [Make sure the milk is added first!]
2. Add the other ingredients.
3. Blend well.
4. Drink right away while chilled, or take with you in a container to drink throughout the day.

Eggs

- ★ Gourmet Scrambled Eggs

- ★ French Toast

- ★ Fresh Vegetable Omelet

- ★ Toad in the Hole

- ★ Curried Egg and Lettuce Sandwiches

Gourmet Scrambled Eggs

B L D

10 minutes to make
Serves 2 adults

Ingredients
6 large eggs
2 teaspoons freshly chopped parsley
½ cup non-fat milk
salt and pepper to taste
2 pieces wholegrain bread for toasting
[only if it's breakfast or lunch]

Method
1. Remove 2 out of 6 yolks.
2. Heat a medium non-stick frying pan and add all the ingredients. Stir occasionally.
3. When the eggs are nearly cooked, remove from the heat, stirring from the base of the pan.
4. Serve immediately on hot, unbuttered toast [no toast if eating for dinner]

Note If you accidentally cook the eggs right through, add another whole egg and mix quickly through the scrambled eggs. This should make them nice and creamy again.

French Toast

B L D

5 minutes to make
Serves 2 adults

Ingredients
4 slices wholegrain bread
4 large eggs
2 tablespoons nonfat milk
salt and pepper to taste
1 tomato or sugar free syrup

Method
1. In a medium bowl, whisk the eggs, milk, salt and pepper.
2. Briefly soak each slice of bread in the egg mixture.
3. Heat a large non-stick frying pan. Place the soaked bread in pan.
4. When browned, turn the bread over.
5. When both sides are browned, serve with grilled tomatoes and, or, sugar free syrup.
6. Serve with scrambled eggs for your portion of protein.

Fresh Vegetable Omelet

B L D

10 minutes to make
Serves 1 adult

Ingredients
4 large eggs [2 yolks only]
2 teaspoons parsley, freshly chopped
1 teaspoon fat free vegetable stock powder
1 small tomato, chopped
½ small onion, chopped
½ cup spring onions, chopped
1 cup crunchy vegetables, freshly chopped
salt and pepper to taste

Method
1. Beat eggs well in a medium mixing bowl.
2. Add remaining ingredients.
3. Heat a medium non-stick frying pan and add the mixture.
4. When the base is cooked and coming away from the sides of the pan, remove the omelet from the stove and place under a preheated griller until the mixture is well cooked and lightly browned on top.
5. Remove the omelet carefully by folding one half on top of the other, then sliding it onto a warmed plate.
6. Serve with a crunchy garden salad.

Toad in the Hole

B L D

15 minutes to make
Serves 1 adult

Ingredients
2 large eggs
1 teaspoon parsley, freshly chopped
salt and pepper to taste
2 slices wholegrain bread
1 ripe tomato

Method
1. In a small mixing bowl, beat 1 egg and add the parsley, salt and pepper.
2. Cut out a small square in the middle of each slice of bread – the size of an egg yolk.
3. Dip the bread in the egg mixture.
4. Heat a large non-stick frying pan and add the bread.
5. Crack 1 egg into the middle of each slice of bread.
6. Place a lid on the pan, and as soon as the bottom of the bread is browned, carefully turn over.
7. Depending on whether you like your eggs runny or hard, remove accordingly.
8. Serve hot with grilled tomatoes, fresh parsley, salt and pepper.

Curried Egg and Lettuce Sandwiches

B L D

☺ ☺ ☹

15 minutes to make
Serves 2 adults

Ingredients
3 large eggs
4 slices of wholegrain bread
1 teaspoon curry powder
2 teaspoons tomato sauce
1 tablespoon non-fat milk [plus a little extra if required]
1 tablespoon fat free salad dressing
1 teaspoon parsley, freshly chopped
salt and pepper to taste
lettuce

Method
1. In a small saucepan, hard boil the eggs.
2. Remove when cooked [approximately 10 minutes], and peel shell under cold water.
3. In a small mixing bowl, place the eggs and other ingredients.
4. Mix thoroughly until nice and creamy, adding extra milk if necessary.
5. Chop the lettuce finely.
6. Spoon egg mixture onto bread and sprinkle lettuce on top.
7. Cut sandwiches into fingers and serve with a garnish of fresh parsley.

Fish

★   Barbequed Salmon with Garlic & Green Onions

★   Grilled Fish with Lemon and Herbs

★   Baked Fish with Tomato Seasoning

★   Red Salmon Salad

★   Tuna Chowder

Barbequed Salmon With Garlic & Green Onions

B L D

15 minutes to make
Serves 4 adults

Ingredients
4 x 5-7oz fillets of fresh salmon
2 teaspoons fresh crushed garlic
8 stalks fresh green onions chopped
1 tablespoon olive oil
2 fresh lemons
4 cups shredded broccoli
1 cup shredded carrots
salt and pepper to taste

Method
1. Heat the barbeque [or skillet] on high
2. Place the salmon onto a foil tray.
3. Rub in garlic, sprinkle chopped green onions, drizzle olive oil, then add salt and pepper to taste.
4. Cook uncovered for 5-10 minutes then turn and cook on the other side.
5. Serve hot or cold with shredded broccoli and carrots, and fresh lemon.

Grilled Fish with Lemon and Herbs

B L D

 ☺ ☺

45 minutes to make
Serves 4 adults

Ingredients
4 x 7oz fresh white fish fillets, 1 inch thick each fillet
2 fresh lemons
salt and pepper to taste
fresh or dried mixed herbs

Method
1. Place the freshly washed fish fillets into a foil tray.
2. Sprinkle with fresh or dried mixed herbs.
3. Add salt and pepper to taste.
4. Squeeze 2 fresh lemons over the fish.
5. Grill for 5 minutes each side.
6. Serve with your favorite non-starch salad and fat free dressing.

Baked Fish with Tomato Seasoning

B L D

45 minutes to make
Serves 4 adults

Ingredients
1 large fresh white fish [gutted and scaled]
1 large tomato
1 large onion
1 lemon
2 spring onion stalks
1 tablespoon salt

Method
1. Wash the fish thoroughly and place on a large sheet of foil [big enough to fold over].
2. Slice the tomato, onion and lemon in circles.
3. Chop the spring onions [not too finely].
4. Spread the ingredients on top of the fish. Add salt.
5. Wrap foil over the fish and bake for approximately 30 minutes at 350°F [180°C].
6. Serve with your favorite non-starch salad and fat free dressing.

Red Salmon Salad

B L D
☹ ☺ ☺

10 minutes to make
Serves 4 adults

Ingredients
2 large cans of red salmon, drained well
1 small onion, finely chopped
1 tablespoon parsley, freshly chopped
2 medium carrots, roughly chopped
2 large celery stalks, roughly chopped
½ a red or green [or both] peppers, roughly chopped
¼ cup lemon juice fat free French or Italian salad dressing
salt and pepper to taste

Method
1. Place all ingredients in a large mixing bowl and mix thoroughly.
2. Serve either hot or cold over half a cup of brown rice or with a dry-baked jacket potato [only if you're eating this for lunch]. You can serve it with a green salad for early dinner.

Tuna Chowder

B L D

40 minutes to make
Serves at least 4 adults

Ingredients

2 large cans of tuna in brine or spring water
[drain one can only]
2 celery stalks, diced
1 medium onion, diced
1 large potato, diced [leave the skin on]
8 mushrooms, sliced
1 teaspoon fresh dill
4 cups fat free chicken stock
1 small can evaporated skim milk
salt and pepper to taste

Method

1. In a large saucepan, combine all the ingredients.
2. Bring to the boil, then reduce the heat. Put a lid on the saucepan and simmer for approximately 30 minutes, stirring occasionally.
3. Serve either hot or cold over half a cup of brown rice or with a dry-baked jacket potato [only if you're eating this for lunch]. You can serve it with a green salad for early dinner.

Chicken

★   Honey Chicken

★   Lime, Chilli & Cilantro Chicken

★   Lemon Herb Chicken

★   Chicken in Homemade Barbecue Sauce

★   Teriyaki Chicken Bowl

255 Body & Soul by Dianne Wilson

Honey Chicken

B L D

😐 ☺ ☺

20 minutes to make
Serves at least 4 adults

Ingredients
2 cups cooked brown rice
6 large chicken breast fillets [skinless and boneless]
1 large onion, chopped
1 cup fat free chicken stock
1 tablespoon parsley, freshly chopped
4 tablespoons honey

Method
1. Chop the chicken into large, bite-sized pieces.
2. In a large non-stick frying pan, cook the chicken, onion, stock, parsley and honey on medium-high heat until chicken is brown.
3. Reduce temperature and remove lid. Cook until sauce thickens slightly [a hot toffee-like consistency].
4. Turn stove off. Add a little water if sauce is too thick, and cover pan with lid.
5. Serve honey chicken with half a cup of brown rice with a side serving of lightly steamed broccoli and carrots. [No rice if you're eating this meal in the evening – serve with a crunchy green salad instead.]

Lime, Chili & Cilantro Chicken   B L D

25 minutes to make [plus one hour to marinade]
Serves 4 adults

Ingredients
4 large chicken breast fillets [skinless and boneless]
2 fresh limes squeezed
½ cup freshly chopped cilantro
1 tablespoon olive oil
1 tablespoon fresh red chili paste
salt and pepper to taste

Method
1. Wash chicken and remove any traces of fat, and cut each breast in half.
2. Prep are 2 sheets of greaseproof paper.
3. Mix the lime, chilli and cilantro, chicken, olive oil, salt and pepper in a bowl and marinade for an hour.
4. Grill the chicken on an outdoor barbeque or indoor grill
5. Serve with crunchy salad vegetables. Garnish with a slice of lime.

Lemon Herb Chicken

B L D

15 minutes to make
Serves 4 adults

Ingredients

4 large chicken breast fillets [skinless and boneless]
2 teaspoons dried mixed herbs
½ cup fat free chicken stock
2 lemons
salt and pepper to taste

Method

1. Wash chicken and leave it in whole fillets.
2. Place in medium-sized non-stick frying pan.
3. Add herbs, the juice of 1½ lemons, stock, pepper and salt.
4. Begin to cook at a medium–high temperature.
5. Place a lid on the saucepan after one side of chicken has been seared and turned over. Reduce heat slightly.
6. After a few minutes the chicken will be cooked [be careful not to overcook and dry out]. Add a little more lemon if necessary.
7. Serve with a wedge of lemon and a fresh garden salad.

Chicken in Homemade Barbecue Sauce

B L D

60 minutes to make
Serves 4–6 adults

Ingredients

6 half chicken breast fillets
pepper to taste
3 teaspoons fat free chicken stock powder
1 medium onion, finely chopped
¼ cup cold water
5 tablespoons white wine
5 tablespoons soy sauce
1 heaped tablespoon tomato purée
1 heaped teaspoon mustard powder
1 teaspoon crushed garlic

Method

1. Preheat oven to 200°C [400°F].
2. Wash and dry fillets very well and slice in half. Rub each piece all over with pepper and some of the stock.
3. Place chicken into a shallow roasting pan, tucking the onion among the pieces. Sprinkle them with the remaining stock and a few drops of water.
4. Place the pan on the highest oven shelf. Cook for 30 minutes.
5. Whisk sauce ingredients until blended, then pour over the chicken. Cook for a further 25 minutes, basting frequently. Serve with a leafy garden salad [no rice if eating this meal for dinner]

Chicken Cordon Bleu

B L D

25 minutes to make
Serves 4 adults

Ingredients
4 large chicken breast fillets [skinless and boneless]
2 large slices low fat smoked ham
2 slices low fat cheese
8 toothpicks
½ cup fat free chicken stock
salt and pepper to taste

Method
1. Wash chicken and remove any traces of fat.
2. Slice chicken in half as you would a bread roll, not quite all the way through.
3. Poke in half a slice of ham and half a slice of cheese.
4. Stitch up along each side with two toothpicks per chicken breast.
5. Heat a large non-stick frying pan and add half the chicken stock.
6. When stock is heated, add the chicken fillets. Keep temperature fairly high until one side is slightly browned.
7. Turn chicken over, place lid on frying pan and reduce heat to low–medium. Add a little more stock if necessary.
8. Serve with steamed winter vegetables and a sprinkle of parsley. [Don't forget – no starchy carbs if you eat this meal in the evening!]

Veal

- ★ Vienna Schnitzel

- ★ Veal Stroganoff

- ★ Italian Veal Casserole

- ★ Cajun Veal Kebabs

- ★ Veal and Broccoli in Creamy Cheese Sauce

Vienna Schnitzel

B L D

☹ ☺ ☹

30 minutes to make
Serves 4 adults

Ingredients
1 cup breadcrumbs
salt and pepper to taste
1 cup cornflour
1 teaspoon sweet paprika
2 eggs
2 tablespoons lemon juice
6 large, very lean veal schnitzel fillets
1 small tube of anchovy paste [optional]
fat free beef gravy powder and water
2 tablespoons lemon juice

Method
1. Prepare 2 sheets of greaseproof paper.
2. Place breadcrumbs with salt mixed in well on one sheet of greaseproof paper, and corn flour, pepper and paprika mixed well on the other.
3. In a small bowl, beat eggs with the lemon juice.
4. Coat the meat in anchovy sauce if using it. Roll meat in the corn flour. Dip it in the egg, then roll in the breadcrumbs.
5. Place the veal in a large, preheated non-stick frying pan.
6. When one side of the meant has browned slightly, turn it over and place a lid on the pan.
7. It will cook quickly so be careful no to overcook. When browned and cooked through, remove from the heat.

Veal Stroganoff

20 minutes to make
Serves 4 adults

Ingredients
2 pounds very lean veal, finely diced
½ cup fat free chicken stock
1 cup button mushrooms
2 packets fat free stroganoff sauce packet mix
1½–2 cups non-fat milk
salt and pepper to taste
2 cups brown or wild rice

Method
1. Lightly brown the veal in the stock in a medium–large non¬stick frying pan. Chop and add the button mushrooms.
2. In a small non-stick saucepan, mix the stroganoff sauce mix with milk until thickened.
3. Pour the sauce into the frying pan. Reduce the sauce if necessary.
4. When the meat and sauce have browned slightly, remove from heat.
5. Serve hot over half a cup of brown or wild rice. [No rice if you eat this dish in the evening.]

Italian Veal Casserole

B L D

☺ ☺ ☺

40 minutes to make
Serves 4 adults

Ingredients
1 medium onion, roughly chopped
1 teaspoon crushed garlic
2 pounds very lean veal, finely diced
½ cup fat free chicken stock
1 cup white wine
1 large can tomatoes, peeled and chopped
1 tablespoon tomato paste
salt and pepper to taste
parsley and lemon rind for garnish

Method
1. In a large non-stick frying pan, cook the onion and garlic in the chicken stock until golden [about 10 minutes].
2. Add the veal and brown slightly on both sides.
3. Pour in wine and let it bubble and reduce a little before adding tomatoes, tomato paste, and salt and pepper.
4. Cover the pan and allow meat to cook slowly for 20 minutes. Remove the lid and let the casserole cook gently for another 10 minutes or until the sauce has reduced.
5. Garnish with chopped parsley and lemon rind and serve with lightly steamed vegetables. [No starchy carbohydrates if you eat this meal in the evening.]

Cajun Veal Kebabs

B L D

30 minutes to make
Serves 4 adults

Ingredients
1 pound lean, bite-sized cubes of veal
2 tablespoons Cajun seasoning
2 tablespoons olive oil
2 large onions
2 large bell peppers, red and green
1 small tin unsweetened pineapple [fresh if available]
1 lemon salt and pepper to taste
12 kebab skewers
2 cups cooked brown or wild rice

Method
1. Marinade the veal in the Cajun seasoning and olive oil for half a day if possible, or for at least one hour.
2. Chop the onion and capsicums into large, bite-sized pieces.
3. Alternatively skewer the veal, onion, pineapple, bell pepper, until skewer is full.
4. Using the same or a little extra Cajun sauce, continue to marinade the kebabs for approximately 20 minutes.
5. If you have the facilities, they are best barbecued. If not, cook in a very hot non-stick frying pan or grill. Ensure that you don't over or undercook.
6. Serve immediately with half a cup of brown or wild rice with a slice of lemon. [Serve without rice if you are eating this dish in the evening.]

Veal and Broccoli in Creamy Cheese Sauce

B L D

20 minutes to make
Serves 4 adults

Ingredients
1 pound very lean veal, finely diced
½ cup fat free chicken stock
salt and pepper to taste
1 medium onion, chopped
2 packets low fat cheese sauce packet mix
1 cup non-fat milk
¼ cup white wine
1 large head of broccoli chopped into small, bite-sized pieces
½ cup green onions, finely chopped

Method
1. In a large non-stick frying pan with lid on, lightly brown the veal in the stock, salt and pepper, white wine, spring onions and onion.
2. In a separate bowl, mix the cheese sauce and milk.
3. When veal is nearly cooked, add the broccoli and simmer for 5 minutes on a low heat with the lid on.
4. Add the cheese sauce mixture and stir well.
5. Allow to simmer for a further 5 minutes and let the cheese sauce go slightly brown.
6. Serve nice and hot over jasmine rice. [No rice if you eat this dish in the evening.]

Beef

★   Satay Beef with Fresh Garden Greens

★   Fillet Steak in Oyster Sauce

★   Pepper Steak with Dijon Mustard and Garlic

★   Beef Curry with Whole Spices

★   Baked Meatloaf with Barbecue Sauce

Satay Beef with Fresh Garden Greens

B   L   D

20 minutes to make
Serves 4 adults

Ingredients

6 fillet steaks, 1 inch thick
1 teaspoon sweet paprika
4 tablespoons satay seasoning
1 teaspoon salt
2 cups fat free beef stock
1 small onion, chopped
1 large head of broccoli, chopped into small, bite-sized pieces

Method

1. Trim the steak of all fat and cut into thin, small strips.
2. Mix the paprika and satay seasoning with the salt.
3. Rub the mixture into the meat thoroughly and leave to marinade for as long as possible.
4. Using a large non-stick frypan on a high heat, place the steak in the pan with half the stock and the onions.
5. When the steak is nearly cooked, add the broccoli.
7. When broccoli has just softened, pour in remaining beef stock
8. Allow to simmer on a low heat for 5 minutes. Add a little water if necessary.

Fillet Steak in Oyster Sauce

B L D

25 minutes to make
Serves 4 adults

Ingredients

6 fillet steaks, 1 inch thick
1 onion, thinly sliced
½ cup fat free beef stock
1 cup bamboo shoots
pepper to taste
4 tablespoons oyster sauce
1 dessertspoon soy sauce
2 cups whole baby green beans
2 cups cooked jasmine rice

Method

1. Remove all fat from steak and cut into thin, bite-sized strips.
2. In a large non-stick frying pan, cook the steak with the onion, stock and pepper.
3. Just before steak is cooked, add the oyster sauce, bamboo shoots, beans and soy sauce.
4. Simmer for 5 minutes on a low heat, being very careful not to overcook.
5. When sauce has reduced slightly, place lid on pan and turn off heat.
6. Serve on a bed of half a cup of jasmine rice with lightly steamed Chinese vegetables. [No rice if you eat this dish in the evening.]

Pepper Steak with Dijon Mustard and Garlic

B L D

25 minutes to make
Serves 4 adults

Ingredients

4 fillet steaks, 1 ½ inches thick
2 tablespoons Dijon seed mustard
1 teaspoon crushed garlic
2 teaspoons pepper
½ teaspoon salt
½ cup thick teriyaki sauce
½ cup water

Method

1. Remove all fat from steak and place into a shallow dish to marinade with all of the other ingredients except the water.
2. In a medium, preheated non-stick frypan, sear the steak both sides then add the rest of the marinade.
3. Reduce the heat and cook until steak is done to taste.
4. Add water a little at a time only if necessary. If necessary, add a little more teriyaki sauce.
5. Serve with thinly-sliced carrots and steamed green vegetables.

Beef Curry with Whole Spices   B L D

30 minutes to make [plus 2 hours simmering time]
Serves 4 adults

Ingredients

2 teaspoons coriander seeds, crushed

1 teaspoon cumin seeds, crushed

1 tablespoon turmeric

1 pound fillet steak, all fat removed, cut into strips

2 large onions, sliced

½ cup fat free beef stock

2 teaspoons crushed garlic

2 fresh capsicums, cut into strips

2 teaspoons ground ginger

½ cup hot water

½ cup low-fat natural yogurt

salt and pepper to taste

Method

1. Place spices in a non-stick frying pan, dry frying for about 5 minutes over a gentle heat.

2. In a separate non-stick frying pan, brown the meat by dry frying and then remove to plate.

3. Add the onions to meat frying pan and cook in beef sock for 5 minutes. Return meat to the pan.

4. Cook for a further 5 minutes. Return meat to the pan.

5. Mix the water and yogurt and add salt. Add to the meat. Cover the frying pan and simmer for 2 hours on a low heat. After 2 hours remove the lid and continue to cook for 15 minutes to reduce the sauce slightly,

Baked Meatloaf with Barbecue Sauce

B L D

 ☺ ☺

60 minutes to make [including baking time]
Serves 4 adults

Ingredients

1 ½ pounds lean beef mince

3 eggs

3 heaped tablespoons corn flour [a little extra if necessary]

2 heaped tablespoons breadcrumbs

4 tablespoons tomato paste

2 tablespoons Worcestershire sauce

2 tablespoons thick fat free teriyaki sauce

1 tablespoon seasoning sauce

1 tablespoon Italian herbs

3 teaspoons dry or 2 stalks of fresh parsley, chopped

1 large onion, chopped finely and

1 large carrot, grated finely

2 teaspoons fat free beef stock powder

2 teaspoons salt and 2 teaspoons pepper

Method

1. Preheat oven to 350°F [180°C]
2. Mix all ingredients except breadcrumbs. If mixture is too wet, keep adding cornflour.
3. Roll mixture in breadcrumbs. Work until mixture sits firm and is well covered. Sprinkle with salt and pepper.
4. Place the meatloaf on a rack and put the rack in a pan. Cover with foil. Cook in the oven [middle shelf] for 25 minutes.

Baked Meatloaf with
Barbecue Sauce
continued

5. Remove foil and continue cooking for another 25 minutes.
6. Serve with barbecue gravy: 2 tablespoons fat free beef gravy powder, 2 tablespoons tomato sauce, 1 tablespoon Worcestershire sauce and 1 cup of water, stirred in a non-stick pan on a low-medium heat. Add water if necessary.

Lamb

★   Roast Lamb with Rosemary

★   Oriental Lamb

★   Irish Stew

★   Lamb Curry

★   Lebanese Green Bean Stew

Roast Lamb with Rosemary   B L D

  ☺

2 ½ hours to make [including baking time]
Serves at least 4 adults

Ingredients
1 medium lean leg of lamb
4 teaspoons 100% fruit strawberry jam
2 tablespoons fresh rosemary leaves
6 bay leaves
2 teaspoons salt and 1 teaspoon pepper
6 medium potatoes
1 large sweet potato
1 large parsnip

Method
1. Preheat the oven to 350°F [180°C]
2. Place lamb in roasting dish with no oil. Spread jam over the leg. Then sprinkle with rosemary, bay leaves, salt and pepper.
3. Cook for an hour with the lid on [or less time for pink meat]. Then in two separate baking dishes, spread out the washed, peeled and cut vegetables, also in no oil.
4. Cook for 20 minutes uncovered.
5. Add veggies to lamb. Continue cooking lamb and veggies, uncovered, for 20 minutes. Remove lamb when brown and crisp. Turn veggies over.
6. Turn oven to 425°F [220°C], to brown veggies. Turn when brown.
7. Serve with honey carrots, boiled peas, fat free beef gravy [no pan juices!] and a side salad.

Oriental Lamb

B L D

☹ ☺ ☺

40 minutes to make
Serves 4 adults

Ingredients

1 pound very lean strips of lamb [fillet is good]
1 large onion, finely sliced
½ cup celery, sliced
2 tablespoons water
1 cup mushrooms, sliced
2 tablespoons soy sauce
5 teaspoons corn flour
1 large clove garlic, crushed
1 cup cherry tomatoes
2 cups snow peas
½ teaspoon fat free beef stock powder

Method

1. Using a large preheated non-stick frypan, sear the lamb then remove from heat and place onto a dish.
2. In a large saucepan, add onion, celery and water and cook on high for 10 minutes.
3. Add lamb and remaining ingredients except tomatoes and snow peas. Stir in gently. Cover with a lid and simmer until meat has cooked [10 more mins]
5. Add snow peas and tomatoes. Cook for 5–7 minutes.
6. Drain off 1 cup of liquid into a small saucepan. Cook on high for approximately 5 minutes. Put all other ingredients in a container with the meat, ready for serving. Pour the sauce over the lamb and vegetables.

Irish Stew

B L D

2 hours to make [including 1½ hours simmering time]
Serves at least 4 adults

Ingredients
2 tablespoons plain flour
2 teaspoons chicken salt
2 pounds lean filleted lamb
1 large onion, sliced
2 large carrots, sliced
2 medium leeks, washed and sliced
salt and pepper to taste
1 large potato, peeled and sliced
1 tablespoon barley
45 oz hot water

Method
1. Mix flour with chicken salt. Dip the meat in the mixture.
2. Put a layer of meat in the bottom of a large non-stick pan, with some of the onions, carrots, leeks and potatoes. Season with salt and pepper.
3. Add more meat and continue layering the ingredients until everything is in.
4. Sprinkle the barley and pour the hot water over it. Bring to simmering point. Spoon off any 'scum' that rises to the surface, then cover the pan with a lid, reduce heat and leave to simmer for 2 hours.
5. When the stew is ready, remove the meat and veggies onto a large, warm serving dish, making sure you leave all the liquid in the pan.

Lamb Curry

B L D

☺ ☺ ☺

40 minutes to make [including simmering time]
Serves at least 4 adults

Ingredients

2 cups precooked very lean lamb, cubed
2 medium-sized Granny Smith apples, peeled, cored and finely sliced
1 small can peeled whole tomatoes
4 teaspoons chutney
2 teaspoons tomato sauce
2 teaspoons Worcestershire sauce
1 teaspoon lemon juice
½ teaspoon lemon rind, finely grated
2 teaspoons curry powder
½ cup fat free beef stock
2 cups cooked jasmine rice [dinner only]
4 cups broccoli cooked – serve on side

Method

1. Place all ingredients except the beef gravy powder and water into a large non-stick frying pan.
2. Simmer on low–medium heat with a lid on for 30 minutes.
3. In a separate bowl, mix the beef gravy powder and water, then pour into frying pan, stirring constantly.
4. Replace lid and continue to simmer for another 5 minutes.
5. Serve with half a cup of jasmine rice for lunch, or with a side salad if you are eating this meal for dinner.

Lebanese Green Bean Stew

B L D

 ☺ ☺

2½ hours to make [including simmering time]
Serves at least 4 adults

Ingredients

½ pound green string beans
1 pound very lean lamb, cubed
several meat bones [no fat]
1½ cups onions, chopped
1½ teaspoons salt
½ teaspoon pepper
½ teaspoon mixed spices
2 tablespoons tomato paste blended with 2½ cups water
2 cloves garlic
1 teaspoon ground coriander

Method

1. String the beans. Leave whole or slice down the center.
2. In a large non-stick frying pan, simmer the meat, bones and onions.
3. Mix in the beans and fry for a few minutes.
4. Add the salt, pepper and mixed spices, then pour in the tomato paste blended with water.
5. Bring to the boil, cover and simmer slowly until the meat is very tender.
6. Crush the garlic with a pinch of salt and the coriander, and cook lightly in a small non-stick frying pan, adding a sprinkle of water to stop any sticking. Cook until garlic smells sweet and stir this mixture into the cooked stew. Serve with freshly steamed broccoli and carrots.

Pork

★   Sweet and Sour Pork

★   Spicy Grilled Pork

★   Pork in Black Bean Sauce

★   Italian Marinated Pork

★   Pork Chow Mein

Sweet and Sour Pork

B L D

40 minutes to make
Serves 4 adults

Ingredients

1 pound very lean fillet of pork, cut into strips
1 large can unsweetened pineapple pieces [drain
and keep juice]
1 cup bamboo shoots [optional]
1 large red pepper, chopped
2 sticks celery, chopped
½ cup water
¼ cup white wine
2 tablespoons tomato sauce
1 tablespoon corn flour
½ cup green onions, chopped

Method

1. Sear the pork in a large non-stick frying pan until just golden, then put aside.
2. Using a large saucepan, add all the ingredients except the corn flour, pineapple juice and bamboo shoots.
3. In a separate bowl, dissolve the corn flour in the pineapple juice, then add to the saucepan.
4. Half-cook the contents of the saucepan on medium heat.
5. Add the pork and the bamboo shoots and cook for a further 10 minutes with the lid on.
6. Serve over half a cup of fluffy rice for lunch or on its own if you're eating this meal for dinner.

Spicy Grilled Pork

B L D

☹ ☺ ☺

30 minutes to make
[also has to be refrigerated overnight]
Serves at least 4 adults

Ingredients
2 cups natural low-fat yogurt
¼ cup French mustard
pinch ground allspice
salt and pepper to taste
1 pound very lean pork fillet, cubed
6 metal or 6 wooden skewers
[soaked for at least 2 hours in water]

Method
1. In a large bowl combine half the yogurt with the mustard and seasonings.
2. Add meat and stir well until thoroughly coated. Cover and refrigerate overnight.
3. Thread meat onto 6 skewers and grill for 15–20 minutes.
4. In a saucepan blend the remaining yogurt with leftover marinade and heat gently. Make sure it doesn't boil.
5. Serve kebabs on a bed of boiled rice, covered with the yogurt sauce. If you're eating this meal for dinner, omit the rice and serve with the sauce and a salad.

Pork in Black Bean Sauce

B L D
 ☺ ☺

40 minutes to make
Serves at least 4 adults

Ingredients

1 pound very lean fillet of pork, cut into strips
3 cloves garlic, crushed
1 apple, peeled and sliced
1 medium onion, sliced
¼ cup black beans
2 tablespoons soy sauce
1 tablespoon honey
1 tablespoon sherry or dry white wine
½ cup water salt and pepper to taste
2 cups cooked rice

Method

1. Place the pork in a large non-stick frying pan and cook until just brown.
2. Combine all the other ingredients in a large bowl.
3. Pour over the pork and cook with the lid on for a further 30 minutes on low–medium heat.
4. Serve with half a cup of rice if eating for lunch, or with some lightly steamed Asian vegetables for dinner.

Italian Marinated Pork

B L D

☹ ☺ ☺

1 hour to make [including simmering time]
Serves at least 4 adults

Ingredients

1 pound lean pork fillet, uncut
2 large onions, finely grated
1 large clove garlic, crushed
½ cup fat free chicken stock
½ cup dry white wine
4 medium carrots, finely grated
1 cup peas
1 can peeled whole tomatoes, drained
1 teaspoon oregano salt and pepper to taste

Method

1. In a large non-stick frying pan with the lid on, simmer the pork, onions, garlic, stock and wine.
2. After around 20 minutes, when the pork is cooked, lift the pork out onto a dish.
3. Add the other ingredients, except the peas, to the pan juices and simmer for 30 minutes with the lid on.
4. Cut the pork into 1-inch slices and return to the simmering sauce. Add the peas and continue cooking for another 10 minutes.
5. Serve hot with lightly steamed green vegetables.

Pork Chow Mein

B L D

  ☹

45 minutes to make
Serves at least 4 adults

Ingredients

1 pound very lean pork, minced
1 onion, finely chopped
1 cup cooked white rice
2½ cups of water
1 tablespoon fat free chicken stock powder
½ cup rice noodles, no oil
1 tablespoon curry powder
¼ cup finely chopped spring onions
4 cups finely shredded cabbage
1 large can tin pineapple pieces, drained
¼ cup freshly chopped chives

Method

1. Combine all the ingredients except the cabbage, pineapple and chives, in a large non-stick frying pan.
2. Stir well until pork is cooked thoroughly, then add the cabbage and pineapple.
3. Cook for a further 15 minutes or so, or until the noodles and all other ingredients are soft. Sprinkle chives on top.
4. Serve hot in a large lettuce cup.

Vegetarian

★   Vegetable Soup

★   Stuffed Zucchini

★   Lentil and Vegetable Moussaka

★   Vegetarian Shepherd's Pie

★   Rice Pilaf

Vegetable Soup

B L D

2 hours to make [including simmering time]
Serves at least 4 adults

Ingredients

1 large onion, chopped

1 large clove garlic, crushed

2 tablespoons soy sauce

1 cup lentils

4 cups water

2 teaspoons fat free chicken stock powder

3 medium carrots, chopped

2 celery stalks, chopped

1 cup cauliflower

2 teaspoons fresh coriander, chopped

salt and pepper to taste

2 teaspoons curry powder [or to taste]

1 cup evaporated non-fat milk

Method

1. In a large saucepan, sauté the onion and garlic in soy sauce.
2. Soak the lentils in water for 10 minutes.
3. Add all ingredients except curry powder and evaporated milk.
4. Simmer for 90 minutes on a very low heat.
5. When completely mushy, blend.
6. Add evaporated milk, curry powder and coriander.
7. Serve piping hot with crunchy side salad. Add a bread roll if you're eating this meal for lunch.

Stuffed Zucchini

B L D

☹ ☺ ☺

60 minutes to make
Serves 4 adults

Ingredients
4 large zucchini
½ cup fat free vegetable stock
1 cup finely chopped mushrooms
1 medium onion, roughly chopped
2 medium tomatoes, roughly chopped
1 celery stalk, sliced
½ teaspoon sweet paprika
salt and pepper to taste

Method
1. Slice the zucchini in half lengthways and scoop out the seeds and flesh.
2. In a large non-stick frying pan, heat the stock until simmering. Add the mushrooms and cook until lightly browned.
3. Add the remaining ingredients and simmer for 5 minutes.
4. Spoon the mixture into the zucchini shells and place them on a non-stick baking tray. 5 Bake at 400°F [200°C] for 45 minutes, or until tender.

Lentil and Vegetable Moussaka   B L D

60 minutes to make
Serves 4 adults

Ingredients
2 oz whole green or brown lentils
2 cups water
1 medium eggplant, cut into small cubes
1½ cups fat free vegetable stock
1 large onion, finely chopped
4 oz red bell pepper, finely chopped
1 large clove garlic, crushed
4 tablespoons red wine
1 tablespoon tomato purée
¼ teaspoon ground cinnamon
2 teaspoons chopped parsley
salt and pepper to taste
For the Topping:
2 eggs [only 1 yolk]
4 tablespoons natural, low-fat yogurt
2 teaspoons grated parmesan cheese
¼ teaspoon ground nutmeg

Method
1. Soften the lentils in the water [no salt].
2. Preheat the oven to 350°F [180°C].
3. Prepare the eggplant cubes. Place them in a colander, sprinkle them with salt and cover with a plate weighed down with a heavy object. Leave them to bleed for 20 minutes or so, then rinse and squeeze them dry in a clean tea towel.

Lentil and Vegetable Moussaka
[continued]

4. Pour half the stock into a medium-sized non-stick frypan and cook the onion and bell pepper until softened [around 10 minutes].
5. Remove them and place on a plate.
6. Using the remaining stock, cook the eggplant in the same frypan. It will take around 10 minutes to soften.
7. Add the bell pepper, and cook for a minute, then add the onion and garlic.
8. In a separate bowl, mix the wine and tomato purée with the cinnamon and parsley. Pour this into the vegetable mixture. Stir in the softened lentils, and add salt and pepper.
9. Stir and combine thoroughly, then spoon everything into an ovenproof dish.
10. Beat all the topping ingredients in a separate bowl.
11. Pour topping mixture over the vegetables.
12. Bake in the oven for 30 minutes or until the top is puffy and golden.

Vegetarian Shepherd's Pie

B L D

90 minutes to make
Serves 4 adults

Ingredients

¾ cup whole brown or green lentils
½ cup split green or yellow peas
2½ cups hot water
1 cup fat free vegetable stock
2 celery stalks, chopped
1 medium onion, chopped
2 medium carrots, chopped
½ medium green bell pepper, chopped
1 large clove garlic, crushed
½ teaspoon dried mixed herbs
¼ teaspoon cayenne pepper
salt and pepper to taste
1 small can peeled whole tomatoes
For the Topping:
1 small onion, chopped
½ cup fat free vegetable stock
3 cups boiled potatoes
2 tablespoons non-fat milk
2 teaspoons parmesan cheese, grated

Method

1. Wash then simmer the lentils and split peas in a large, covered saucepan for around 45–60 minutes, or until the peas and lentils have absorbed the water and are soft.
2. Preheat the oven to 375°F [190°C].

Vegetarian Shepherd's Pie
[continued]

3. Simmer the stock in a large non-stick pan. Add the celery, onion, carrots and bell pepper. Cook gently until softened, adding a little more water if necessary.
4. Mash a little. Add to lentil mixture. Then add the garlic, herbs, spices, salt and pepper. Spoon the mixture into a large pie dish. Arrange the sliced tomatoes on top.
5. For the topping, sauté the onion in the stock in a small non-stick frying pan.
6. Mash the potatoes, then add the cooked onion, milk and parmesan cheese, and mix well.
7. Season with salt and pepper, then spread on top of the ingredients in the pie dish.
8. Bake for about 20 minutes or until the top is lightly browned.
9. Serve with some tomato sauce or appropriate chutney and a light crunchy green salad, with a no oil dressing.

Rice Pilaf

B L D

 ☺ ☹

60 minutes to make
Serves 6–8 adults

Ingredients
1¾ cups lentils and water for boiling
2 large onions
½ cup fat free vegetable stock
2 cups rice, washed and drained
1 tablespoon salt
soy sauce to taste

Method
1. Wash the lentils well.
2. Slice onions into fine half-circles.
3. Toss into a hot, medium-sized non-stick frying pan, and keep tossing until golden brown. Splash drops of stock to help the onions brown, but be careful not to add too much water.
4. Remove half the onions from the pan and place on a side plate.
5. In a large saucepan, boil the lentils in water until nearly tender, approximately 20–25 minutes.
6. Mix in the rice and bring back to the boil. Reheat the remaining stock until very hot, then toss in the remaining onions. Pour them onto the lentils and rice.
7. Add salt, cover tightly, turn down the heat and simmer slowly until the rice is tender and all the fluid is absorbed, approximately 20 minutes.
8. Serve hot or cold, garnished with the golden brown onion slices. If served cold, serve with salad greens.

Kids' Meals

Recommended by kids...

★   Hamburgers

★   Macaroni and Cheese

★   Kids' Spaghetti

★   Crumbed Fish Fillets

★   Colorful Chicken Kebabs

Hamburgers

B L D

20 minutes to make
Serves 4 kids

Ingredients
½ pound very lean beef, minced
1 small onion
1 medium tomato some interesting lettuce [raddichio, butter, cos]
4 slices beetroot tomato sauce
4 hamburger buns

Method
1. Heat a large non-stick frying pan on high.
2. Make the mince into four even patties and put them into the pan.
3. Cut the onion into very thin slices, but do not separate rings.
4. Cook them in the pan with the mince.
5. Turn the patties after 5–7 minutes.
6. Split and toast the hamburger buns.
7. When patties are cooked, remove and place neatly on half of the bun. Top with onion rings.
8. Add the salad and tomato sauce.
9. Serve straightaway with Cajun Baked Sweet Potato Chips [see p. 266].

Macaroni and Cheese

B L D

 ☺ ☺

20 minutes to make
Serves 4 kids

Ingredients

2 cups uncooked macaroni elbows or bowties
4 cups water
pinch salt
2 packets low fat cheese sauce packet mix
non-fat milk [as directed on back of the packet, plus a little extra]

Method

1. Using a medium-sized saucepan, cook the macaroni in slightly salted water.
2. In a small non-stick saucepan, mix the cheese sauce with milk as directed on packet.
3. Keep adding milk as you need it. Make sure the sauce isn't too thick.
4. When macaroni is cooked, after 15 minutes, remove from heat, drain and rinse well.
5. Empty macaroni into a dish and pour the cheese sauce over.

Kid's Spaghetti

B L D

60 minutes to make
Serves 4 kids

Ingredients

1/4 packet thin spaghetti noodles [or any other interesting type of pasta]
4 cups water
pinch salt
½ pound very lean beef, minced
1 small tin whole peeled tomatoes [no oil added]
2 teaspoons mixed herbs
1 teaspoon fat free beef stock powder

Method

1. Using a large frying pan, cook the minced beef.
2. Add tomatoes, stock and herbs.
3. Reduce heat to very low, place a lid on the frying pan, and leave simmering for 45 minutes.
4. When the sauce is nearly ready, cook the spaghetti noodles in a large saucepan filled with slightly salty water.
5. When spaghetti is cooked [after 15 minutes], remove from heat, drain and rinse well.
6. Empty into a serving dish. Pour sauce over and mix in.
7. Serve hot with a small, simple salad of lettuce, carrots and tomato, with some Italian bread.

Crumbed Fish Fillets   B L D

☺ ☺ ☺

20 minutes to make
Serves 4 kids

Ingredients
4 medium white fish fillets [as boneless as possible]
1 cup corn flour
1 cup breadcrumbs
2 eggs
salt and pepper to taste
4 small lemon wedges

Method
1. Wash the fillets well.
2. Preheat a large non-stick frying pan on high.
3. Prepare 2 pieces of greaseproof paper, 1 with corn flour, the other with breadcrumbs.
4. Whisk eggs with salt and pepper to taste, in a small bowl.
5. Roll fillets in the cornflour, dip well in the egg mixture then roll straight in the breadcrumbs.
6. Place fillets in the hot frying pan, watching carefully that they don't burn. Reduce the heat immediately, and place the lid on top.
7. After a couple of minutes, turn fillets over very carefully with a spatula and keep cooking until brown.
8. Sprinkle in a little water, for extra moisture, which also helps the fish to brown slightly.
9. Serve hot with some Creamy Mashed Potatoes [see p. 322], steamed fibrous vegetables, and a lemon wedge on the side.

Colorful Chicken Kebabs

B L D

20 minutes to make
Serves 4 kids

Ingredients

½ cup oyster sauce
3 single chicken breast fillets
1 large carrot
2 pineapple rings
½ small green pepper
1 small tomato
8 kebab skewers

Method

1. Wash and trim the chicken of all fat, and cut into bite-sized cubes.
2. Marinate the chicken in the oyster sauce for about 10 minutes.
3. Cut all the fruit and vegetables into bite-sized pieces.
4. Heat a large non-stick frying pan, or a grill or barbeque, on high.
5. Place all the bite-sized pieces, including the chicken, on the kebabs, to make them colorful and fun.
6. When the pan is hot, toss in the kebabs, four at a time. Turn them as they cook.
7. Remove when cooked and serve with a crunchy salad.

Soups

★   Butternut Squash, Parsnip and Tomato

★   Chicken and Corn

★   Leek, Onion and Potato

★   Minestrone

★   Homestyle Beef and Vegetable

Butternut Squash, Parsnip and Tomato Soup

B L D

25 minutes to make
Serves 4 adults

Ingredients

1 medium–large parsnip
½ butternut squash
4 ripe tomatoes
1 teaspoon dried mixed herbs
1 teaspoon fat free vegetable stock powder
salt and pepper to taste
a little low-fat sour cream [only if it's Treat Day]
fresh chives, finely chopped, for garnish

Method

1. Remove skin from butternut squash and parsnip.
2. Chop butternut squash, parsnip and tomatoes into chunks.
3. Steam the butternut squash and parsnip in a large saucepan.
4. When cooked, place all ingredients into a large saucepan with 2 tablespoons of water.
5. Simmer on a low heat until the tomatoes are cooked.
6. Blend all the ingredients until it reaches a soup consistency.
7. If you've been good all week, you may add two teaspoons of low-fat sour cream or yogurt and a sprinkle of chives.

Chicken and Pea Soup

B L D

50 minutes to make
Makes 10–12 servings

Ingredients

6 half chicken breast fillets, finely chopped
10 cups water
1 small onion, roughly chopped
2 slices low fat smoked ham, finely chopped
1 knot root ginger [about 1 inch long], finely chopped
6 large stalks spring onions, finely chopped
2 cups peas
3 tablespoons corn flour
1/3 cup water
2 teaspoons soy sauce
1 egg

Method

1. Place chicken in a large saucepan with the water.
2. Bring to the boil and simmer on a low heat for approximately 40 minutes or until chicken is cooked.
3. Add all other ingredients except corn flour, water, soy sauce and egg. Bring to a boil.
4. In a small container, mix corn flour and water to a smooth paste, add to soup and let simmer, stirring for 3 minutes.
5. Add soy sauce.
6. In a small container, beat the egg lightly with a fork, then stir into the soup.
7. Serve piping hot with a sprinkle of salt and pepper.

Leek, Onion and Potato Soup   B L D

45 minutes to make
Makes 4–6 servings

Ingredients
4 large leeks
2 medium potatoes, peeled and diced
1 medium onion, finely chopped
2 teaspoons fresh chives, finely chopped
1 teaspoon fat free vegetable stock powder
4 cups water
salt and pepper to taste
1 cup non-fat milk

Method
1. Remove outer layer of leeks, chop finely, wash thoroughly and drain well.
2. In a large saucepan, add leeks, potatoes, onion, stock, and half a cup of water. Stir with a wooden spoon so everything is coated with the chicken stock.
3. Add salt and pepper, then cover and let the vegetables sweat over a very low heat for 15 minutes.
4. Add the stock and milk, bring to simmering point, put the lid back on and let the soup simmer very gently for a further 20 minutes or until the vegetables are soft. Be careful not to overheat or boil over.
5. If you don't like chunky soup, use a liquidizer to purée the ingredients.
6. Stir in chopped chives and serve nice and hot with a fresh roll.

Minestrone Soup

B L D

45 minutes to make
Makes 10–12 servings

Ingredients

2 potatoes with the skin on, roughly chopped
4 carrots, peeled and finely sliced
3 onions, roughly chopped
1 teaspoon crushed garlic
1 medium can red kidney beans [no oil]
½ cup fat free chicken stock
14 cups fat free beef stock [6 teaspoons stock and 14 cups hot water]
1 large can peeled tomatoes
4 celery stalks, finely sliced
3 slices low fat smoked ham, roughly chopped
1 cup macaroni
1 tablespoon chopped parsley
1 dessertspoon freshly chopped basil
salt and pepper to taste

Method

1. Sauté the vegetables and ham with the chicken stock in a large saucepan. Add beef stock, beans and tomatoes.
2. Bring to the boil, cover and simmer for 30 minutes.
3. Add macaroni and simmer uncovered, until tender.
4. Serve with a sprinkle of parsley and salt and pepper.

Homestyle Beef and Vegetable   B L D

Make overnight
Makes 10–12 servings

Ingredients

4 cups fat free beef stock
1 cup barley
2 ½ pounds very lean beef, cubed
4 carrots, roughly grated
2 turnips, roughly grated
1 small rutabaga, roughly grated
1 large leek, roughly chopped
1 cup chopped celery
½ cup fresh parsley, finely chopped

Method

1. In a very large cooking pot, place all the ingredients.
2. Cook for 1–1½ hours or until the meat is tender.
3. Leave overnight for fat to set. It will do this best in the fridge.
4. Skim any fat off the top of the soup the next morning.
5. Add more beef stock if necessary, and simmer for another hour, or until barley is nice and soft.
6. Serve piping hot with a leafy green salad.

Salads

★   Italian Tomato

★   Tangy Coleslaw

★   Chinese Greens

★   Waldorf

★   Tabbouleh

Italian Tomato Salad

B L D

10 minutes to make
Serves 2 adults

Ingredients
2 large tomatoes, sliced
2 large zucchini, sliced
1 large yellow onion, sliced
a few fresh basil leaves
salt and pepper to taste
¾ cup fat free Italian dressing

Method
1. Using a glass salad bowl, alternately layer all the vegetables and basil leaves.
2. Pour the salad dressing over everything.
3. Add salt and pepper to taste.
4. Serve on its own or to accompany another dish.

Tangy Coleslaw

B L D

☺ ☺ ☺

15 minutes to make
Serves 4 adults

Ingredients

½ cup carrots, shredded
¼ cup white onion, finely chopped
1 cup mixed red and green cabbage, shredded
2 teaspoons parsley, finely chopped
¼ cup brown vinegar
¼ cup fat free Italian dressing
2 teaspoons honey
pepper to taste

Method

1. Combine vegetables in a large mixing bowl.
2. Mix vinegar, dressing, honey and pepper in a separate, smaller bowl.
3. Pour liquid ingredients over vegetables and mix well.
4. Cover and chill.
5. Serve as an accompaniment to another dish.

Chinese Greens

B L D
 ☺ ☺

10 minutes to make
Serves 4 adults

Ingredients
2 cups chopped Chinese green vegetables
2 cups fresh baby spinach leaves
1 cup fresh bamboo shoots
1 cup thinly sliced radishes
½ cup chopped mushrooms
1 small container cherry tomatoes
¼ cup Italian dressing [no oil]
1 tablespoon honey
2 tablespoons soy sauce
pepper to taste

Method
1. Thoroughly wash and drain all green vegetables, remove all stems, then place in large glass salad bowl.
2. Add radishes, mushrooms, tomatoes and bamboo shoots.
3. Mix dressing, honey, soy sauce and pepper in small bowl.
4. Pour dressing over salad and toss well.

Waldorf Salad

B L D

☹ ☺ ☺

10 minutes to make
Serves 4 adults

Ingredients
1 tablespoon of lemon juice
3 large red apples, washed and diced
1½ cups celery, washed and diced, unstrung
¼ cup raisins
1 low fat vanilla flavored yogurt parsley for garnish

Method
1. Place apples in a medium-sized glass salad bowl.
2. Squeeze lemon juice over apples to prevent discoloring.
3. Add remaining ingredients and toss well.
4. Cover and chill before serving.

Tabbouleh

B L D

1½ hours to make
Serves 4 adults

Ingredients

½ cup instant bulghur [cracked wheat]

8–10 green onions

2 teaspoons salt

¼ teaspoon pepper

¼ teaspoon mixed spices

5 cups very finely chopped parsley

¼ cup very finely chopped fresh mint or 2 teaspoons dried mint

3 large tomatoes, finely chopped

¼ cup lemon juice

¼ cup fat free Mediterranean salad dressing

Method

1. Wash the bulghur and drain well by squeezing out excess water with cupped hands.
2. Place in a bowl and refrigerate for at least 1 hour.
3. Trim the green onions, leaving about ¾ inch of green.
4. Finely chop the white of the spring onions and mix it into the drained burghul with the salt, pepper and spices.
5. Finely chop the green of the green onions and place it with parsley, mint and tomatoes on top of the burghul mixture. Set aside in the refrigerator until ready to serve.
6. Just before serving, add the lemon juice and dressing and toss well. Add salt and lemon juice to taste.

Vegetables

★   Honey Carrots

★   Super Stir Fry

★   Baked Sweet Potatoes with Garlic

★   Barbecued Italian Peppers

★   Ratatouille

Honey Carrots

B L D

15 minutes to make
Serves 4 adults

Ingredients
1 cup water
8 medium carrots, peeled and cut diagonally, ¼ inch thick
¾ teaspoon ground cumin
½ teaspoon fresh ginger, crushed
¼ teaspoon ground coriander
¼ teaspoon cayenne pepper
2 tablespoons honey
2 teaspoons lemon juice

Method
1. Using a medium-sized saucepan, boil water.
2. When boiling, add everything except honey and lemon juice.
3. Reduce the heat and simmer for 5 minutes.
4. Add lemon juice and honey.
5. Turn up heat and cook until all liquid has evaporated and carrots are soft [around 5 minutes]. Drain and serve.

Super Stir Fry

B L D

15 minutes to make
Serves 4 adults

Ingredients

1 medium head of broccoli
1 small head cauliflower
½ red pepper
1 cup snow peas
1 large zucchini, sliced in chunks
2 large carrots, finely sliced
1 medium yellow onion, finely sliced
1 cup shredded red and white cabbage
½ cup oyster sauce

Method

1. Wash broccoli and cauliflower and prepare into small, bite-sized pieces.
2. Preheat a large non-stick frying pan on high then add all the ingredients. Cover with lid.
3. Cook for a couple of minutes, and stir well.
4. After another 5 minutes with the lid on, remove from heat and serve.

Baked Sweet Potatoes with Garlic B L D

60 minutes to make
Serves 4 adults

Ingredients
2 large sweet potatoes, washed and peeled
¼ cup finely chopped onion
2 tablespoons garlic crushed
2 tablespoons olive oil
salt and pepper to taste

Method
1. Pre-heat oven to 425°F [220°C]
2. Chop the sweet potatoes into bite sizes pieces.
3. Sprinkle over the onion, crushed garlic and drizzle with olive oil.
4. Grind salt and pepper to taste.

Barbequed Italian Peppers

B L D

20 minutes to make
Serves 4 adults

Ingredients

4 large red peppers, washed
1 cup red wine vinegar
2 tablespoons fresh basil, chopped
salt and pepper to taste

Method

1. Preheat an outdoor barbeque or an indoor health grill until very hot.
2. Place peppers on grill and turn. Continue turning until skin has blistered and blackened on all sides.
3. Remove and place in a bowl of cold salty water to loosen skins. Carefully remove skins.
4. After removing skins, place in a shallow serving dish.
5. Pour over vinegar, salt and pepper, and sprinkle with basil.
6. Cover and chill.

Ratatouille

B L D

  ☺

30 minutes to make
Serves 4 adults

Ingredients
2 large eggplants
3 medium zucchini
1 red and 1 green pepper, cored, deseeded and chopped
1 large can whole peeled tomatoes [no oil], chopped
1 tablespoon fresh basil or 2 teaspoons dried basil
¾ cup fat free vegetable stock
2 large cloves garlic, crushed
2 medium onions, roughly chopped
salt and pepper to taste
fresh basil leaves or parsley to garnish

Method
1. Wipe eggplant and zucchini, cut into 1 inch slices, then halve each slice.
3. Put eggplant and zucchini into a colander. Sprinkle generously with salt. Press them down with a plate. Let stand for 1 hour.
4. In a medium non-stick frying pan, heat the stock. Add onion and garlic. Cook for 10 minutes then add green pepper.
5. Dry zucchini and eggplant in a towel, then add to the pan and add the basil, salt and pepper. Stir once very well. Simmer gently with the lid on for about 30 minutes.
6. Add the tomato. Taste and season. Cook for 10 minutes or so more with the lid off.

Potatoes

★   Summer Potato Salad

★   Cajun Baked Sweet Potato Chips

★   Potatoes au Gratin

★   Chipped Potato Grits

★   Creamy Mashed Potatoes

Summer Potato Salad

B L D

30 minutes to make
Serves 4 adults

Ingredients

2½ pounds red potatoes, washed and cut into small cubes
[leave skin on]

4 eggs, boiled and roughly chopped

½ cup finely chopped fresh parsley

½ cup finely chopped fresh chives

1 large stalk of celery, finely chopped

1 large onion, finely chopped

1 cup low-fat natural yogurt

2 tablespoons fat free Italian salad dressing

2 tablespoons fat free mayonnaise

1 teaspoon mustard powder

½ teaspoon salt

½ teaspoon pepper

Method

1. Parboil the potatoes, being careful not to cook them until
   they're mushy.
2. Combine all the other ingredients in a mixing bowl and
   stir well.
3. Place potatoes in a serving dish and add the dressing.
4. Mix and refrigerate.
5. Best served cold.

Cajun Baked Sweet Potato Chips   B L D

30 minutes to make
Serves 4 adults

Ingredients
2½ pounds sweet potatoes, washed and cut into chip strips
[or substitute red potatoes with skin left on]
3 eggs
salt and pepper to taste
1 small jar Cajun spices

Method
1. Preheat oven to 425°F [220°C].
2. Beat eggs with salt, pepper and Cajun spices.
3. Dip potato chip strips in egg mixture then place on a non-stick tray and place in the oven to bake for 15 minutes.
4. Check them. When they're brown on one side, turn them, adding a little more Cajun spices and salt.
5. When they're cooked through, after about another 15 minutes, remove from oven.
6. Serve and eat right away.

Potatoes au Gratin

B L D

60 minutes to make
Serves 4 adults

Ingredients

2½ pounds red potatoes, washed and cut into very thin slices [leave skin on]
2 extra-large onions, cut into fine rings
¼ cup finely chopped fresh spring onions
1 packet fat free cheese sauce mix
3 cups non-fat milk
4 slices low fat ham, finely chopped
salt and pepper to taste
1 teaspoon sweet paprika
½ teaspoon crushed garlic

Method

1. Preheat the oven to 425°F [220°C].
2. In a large, ovenproof casserole dish, place the potato slices and onion rings and mix well with the ham and spring onions.
3. Mix cheese sauce, milk, and other ingredients in a separate bowl.
4. Pour sauce over the potato mixture.
5. Place in the oven until potatoes are browned slightly and soft, approximately 60 minutes.

Chipped Potato Grits

B L D

20 minutes to make
Serves 4 adults

Ingredients

2½ pounds red potatoes, washed and cut into very thin slices [leave skin on]
2 extra-large onions, cut into fine rings
1 teaspoon dried dill
2 cups fat free vegetable stock

Method

1. Place all ingredients in a large non-stick frying pan and cover.
2. Allow to cook on a medium-high heat until potatoes are soft.
3. Reduce the heat and allow to simmer while fluids reduce.
4. Add a little water as you go if necessary.
5. Stir so it looks really messy.

Creamy Mashed Potatoes

B L D

Large Starchy Carbohydrate
15 minutes to make
Serves 4 adults

Ingredients

2½ pounds red potatoes, cut into quarters
[leave skin on]
1 egg
a little non-fat milk
salt and pepper to taste
¼ cup freshly chopped parsley

Method

1. Boil the potatoes until soft.
2. Drain well and place in bowl ready for mixing.
3. In a separate bowl, whisk the egg.
4. Mash the potatoes dry at first, adding the egg. Then, using an electric mixer, give the potatoes a good mash.
5. Add a little skim milk until the mixture is nice and creamy. Be careful not to add too much. If you do, put in a saucepan on the stove on medium heat until reduced a little.
6. Add salt and pepper to taste and garnish with parsley.

Pasta

★   Spaghetti Bolognaise

★   Fettucine Boscaiola

★   Fettucine Salmone

★   Gnocchi with Crabmeat

★   Tortellini with Chicken and Mushrooms

Spaghetti Bolognaise

B L D

20 minutes to make
Serves at least 4 adults

Ingredients

1 packet spaghetti and water for boiling

1 pound lean beef mince

1 medium onion, chopped

1 cup fat free beef stock

¼ cup red wine

4 teaspoons dried Italian herbs

1 teaspoon crushed garlic

2 tablespoons fat free beef gravy powder

1 cup water

1 cup tomato paste

2 cups tomato soup

2 cups whole peeled tomatoes

Method

1. Cook spaghetti in a large saucepan of boiling water, stirring occasionally. Add more water if necessary.
2. In a large non-stick frying pan, cook the beef, onion, stock and wine on medium–high heat until brown.
3. Turn down heat and add herbs, garlic, tomato paste, tomato puree and whole tomatoes. Stir.
4. In a separate bowl, mix the beef gravy powder with 1 cup of water and slowly add to the other ingredients.
5. Turn off stove and cover frying pan with a lid.
6. Drain spaghetti and wash thoroughly using a colander.
7. Serve bolognaise sauce on spaghetti piping hot, with a side serve of salad vegetables.

Fettuccine Boscaiola

B L D

😐 ☺ 🙁

25 minutes to make
Serves at least 4 adults

Ingredients
1 large packet fettuccine and water for boiling
1 large onion, finely chopped
3 large green onion stalks, finely chopped
4 slices low fat smoked ham, finely chopped
1 cup button mushrooms, finely chopped
½ cup fat free chicken stock
1 teaspoon dried or fresh parsley
salt and pepper to taste
2 packets low fat cheese sauce packet mix
3 cups non-fat milk

Method
1. Cook fettuccine in a large saucepan of boiling water, stirring occasionally. Add more water if necessary. Remove from stove before noodles become too soft.
2. In a large non-stick frypan, cook onion, green onions, ham, mushrooms, stock and parsley on medium high until browned. Add a little water if necessary. Remove from stove.
3. In a saucepan, add cheese sauce and half the milk.
4. Stir constantly until sauce thickens, then add the remaining milk until it is a pancake-type consistency.
5. Drain and rinse fettuccine and return to large saucepan.
6. Add ingredients from the frying pan, then add cheese sauce. Mix well and transfer to container for serving.
7. Allow to sit. Add more milk, if necessary, as sauce thickens. Serve hot with a leafy green salad.

Linguine Salmone

B L D

  ☹

25 minutes to make
Serves at least 4 adults

Ingredients

1 large packet linguine and water for boiling
1 large onion, finely chopped
3 large green onion stalks, finely chopped
4 slices low fat smoked ham, chopped
½ cup fat free chicken stock
2 packets low fat cheese sauce packet mix
1 teaspoon dried or fresh parsley
1 teaspoon Italian herbs
1 teaspoon pepper
pinch of salt
5 oz smoked salmon, cut into thin strips
½ cup fat free thousand island dressing
2 tablespoons tomato sauce
1 cup button mushrooms, finely chopped
3 cups skim milk

Method

1. Cook linguine in a large saucepan of boiling water, stirring occasionally. Add more water if necessary. Remove from stove before noodles are too soft.
2. In a large non-stick frypan, cook the onion, green onions, ham, mushrooms, stock and parsley on medium–high until browned. Add a little water if necessary. Remove from the stove.

Linguine Salmone
[continued]

3. Pour the cheese sauce mix and half of the milk into a small non-stick saucepan.
4. Stir constantly until sauce thickens, then add the remaining milk until a pancake-type consistency is reached.
5. Drain and rinse fettuccine and return to large saucepan.
6. Add the ingredients from the frypan. Add the cheese sauce, salmon, dressing, tomato sauce and mixed herbs.
7. Mix well and transfer to a container for serving.
8. Allow to sit. Add more milk if necessary as starch begins to thicken sauce.
9. Serve piping hot with a leafy green salad.

Gnocchi with Crabmeat

B L D

25 minutes to make
Serves at least 4 adults

Ingredients

1 packet fresh potato gnocchi
1 packet low fat cheese sauce packet mix
2 cups non-fat milk
pinch salt
1 teaspoon pepper
1 large can white crabmeat [fresh if available]
1 teaspoon dried or fresh parsley

Method

1. Boil water in a large saucepan, then add the gnocchi. Cook for 5 minutes on high. Ensure you don't overcook. Drain then wash with cold water.
2. In a small non-stick saucepan, add the cheese sauce mix, milk, salt and pepper.
3. Stir constantly until sauce thickens, adding more milk if necessary.
4. Add the crabmeat to the cooked and thickened cheese sauce, stirring well.
5. Place the gnocchi in a serving dish. Pour the crabmeat and cheese sauce over gnocchi and mix well.
6. Allow to sit. Add more milk if necessary as starch begins to thicken.
7. Garnish with parsley and serve piping hot.

Tortellini with Chicken and Mushrooms

B L D

25 minutes to make
Serves at least 4 adults

Ingredients
1 packet fresh low fat tortellini
6 half chicken breast fillets, cut into bite-sized pieces
1 medium onion, finely chopped
4 large fresh spring onion stalks, finely chopped
4 slices low fat smoked ham
½ cup fat free chicken stock
1 teaspoon dried or fresh parsley
2 teaspoons Dijon seed mustard
1 cup button mushrooms, finely chopped
1 teaspoon pepper
large pinch salt
1 packet low fat cheese sauce packet mix
1 packet fat free stroganoff sauce mix
3 cups non-fat milk

Method
1. Boil water in a large saucepan. Add pasta, and cook for 5–7 minutes on high. Don't overcook. When you drain pasta, rinse with cold water.
2. In a large non-stick frying pan, cook the chicken, onion, spring onions, ham, mushrooms, stock, parsley and mustard on medium–high until browned. Add a little water if necessary, and remove from the stove.
3. Place the cheese and stroganoff mixes and half of the milk in a small non-stick saucepan.

Tortellini with Chicken and Mushrooms
[continued]

4. Stir constantly until sauce thickens, then add the remaining milk until a pancake-type consistency is reached.
5. Add the sauce and pasta to the large frypan, mixing in well.
6. Once heated through, transfer to a suitable dish for serving.
7. Allow to sit. Add a little more milk if necessary as starch begins to thicken.
8. Serve piping hot with steamed vegetables.

Rice

★   Combination Fried Rice

★   Mexican Rice

★   Rice on the Side

★   Japanese Rice [Chirashi Zushi]

★   Rice Pudding

Combination Fried Rice

B L D

45 minutes to make
Makes 6–8 servings

Ingredients

6 cups cooked white rice [or brown if you prefer]
½ cup fat free chicken stock
4 slices low fat ham, finely chopped
1 large onion, finely chopped
¾ cup finely chopped green onions
2 eggs, beaten
¼ cup soy sauce
salt and pepper to taste

Method

1. In a large non-stick frying pan, add the stock, ham, onion and green onions and cook until brown. Add a little extra stock if necessary.
2. In a small non-stick frying pan, add the eggs with soy sauce, stir to blend and cook as you would an omelet. Chop when cooked.
3. Add rice gradually to frying pan ingredients, stirring through.
4. Add the egg and fold through.
5. Add salt and pepper.
6. Serve piping hot, or cold the next day!

Mexican Rice

B L D

45 minutes to make
Serves 4 adults

Ingredients
1 cup fat free chicken stock
1 small onion, chopped
1 small green bell pepper, chopped
2 cups cooked white or brown rice
½ cup diced tomato
1 cup mild salsa

Method
1. Using a large non-stick frying pan on a medium heat, heat half the stock.
2. Add onion and bell pepper and cook until tender.
3. Add tomato, remaining stock and salsa.
4. Cook until boiling.
5. Stir in cooked rice, cover with lid, turn off heat and leave sitting for 5 minutes.
6. Great served as a side dish with fish or chicken.

Rice on the Side

B L D
  ☹

40 minutes to make
Serves 4

Ingredients
2 cups cooked brown rice
1½ cups peas
2 eggs, beaten
1 small onion, finely chopped
soy sauce to taste pepper to taste

Method
1. Cook rice until soft, then drain and wash well.
2. Into a large serving dish add the rice, mixed with peas.
3. In a small non-stick pan cook the eggs scrambled style, stirring all the time.
4. Add the onion to the egg and mix well.
5. Add the egg and onion to the rice and peas.
6. Pour a little soy sauce and pepper over the mixture and serve either hot or cold.

Japanese Rice
[Chirashi Zushi]

B L D

 😐 ☺ ☹

30 minutes to make
Serves 4

Ingredients
2 cups short-grain white rice
3 cups water
1 small cucumber
1 teaspoon salt
6 teaspoons white vinegar [or rice wine]
3½ teaspoons sugar
5 oz white fish fillet
2 eggs, well beaten
1/2 cup peas, cooked
1 tablespoon shredded preserved ginger
Sauce:
2 tablespoons soy sauce
1 tablespoon white vinegar

Method
1. Wash rice, put into a heavy-based saucepan, cover with water and cook, covered, on low heat until tender. Put aside.
2. Wipe cucumber and rub with a little salt. Shred or grate, then marinate in a mixture of 3 teaspoons vinegar and 1 teaspoon sugar.
3. Steam or boil fish fillet until soft, then flake or chop coarsely. Sprinkle with a mixture of 3 teaspoons vinegar, 1½ teaspoons sugar and ½ teaspoon salt.

Japanese Rice
[Chirashi Zushi]
[continued]

4. Mix eggs with 1 teaspoon sugar and ½ teaspoon salt and pour into large non-stick pan. Cook until firm, turn and cook other side, then remove and cook.
5. When cool, shred with a sharp knife.
6. For the sauce, mix soy sauce with vinegar and pour into rice and mix in with a chopstick, then fold in fish, cucumber, shredded egg and peas.
7. Garnish with shredded ginger.

Rice Pudding

B L D

 ☺

45 minutes to make
Serves 4 adults

Ingredients
1½ cups white or brown rice
2 cups non-fat milk
4 teaspoons 100% fruit jam of your choice
½ cup raisins
½ teaspoon nutmeg
2 teaspoons vanilla essence
2 slices toasted white bread

Method
1. Preheat the oven at 400°F [205°C].
2. Place the rice, milk, fruit, nutmeg and vanilla essence in a casserole dish.
3. Spread the jam over the bread and cut into bite-sized squares.
4. Place pieces of bread over the top of the mixture so it f its like a lid.
5. Bake in the oven until brown and rice is cooked and thickened, approximately 40 minutes.

Desserts

- ★   Chocoholic's Dream

- ★   Berry Delight

- ★   Banana Split

- ★   Honey and Lemon Crêpes

- ★   Srawberries with a Balsamic Reduction

Chocoholic's Dream   B L D
😐 ☺ ☹

10 minutes to make
Serves 4 adults

Ingredients
4 cups fat free chocolate ice-cream
3 cups low-fat vanilla jello
4 teaspoons low-fat chocolate topping
fat free chocolate powder [drink mix]

Method
1. This dessert is best served in either a tall, clear, dessert goblet or a clear bowl.
2. Spoon in the ice-cream, then layer in the jello, then topping. Repeat until the bowl is full.
3. Sprinkle generously with chocolate powder.

Berry Delight

B L D

10 minutes to make
Serves 4 adults

Ingredients
3 cups low-fat vanilla jello
8 teaspoons fat free chocolate powder [drink mix]
4 cups fat free frozen fruit ice-cream
fresh mint for garnish
1 pound fresh mixed berries [or any one alone]

Method
1. This dessert is best served in either a tall clear dessert goblet or a clear bowl.
2. First pour in the jello, evenly distributing it over the four dishes or glasses.
3. Sprinkle 2 teaspoons of chocolate powder over each serving.
4. Tumble in the mixed or single berries, ensuring you fill the dish amply. Do not mix in with the jello.
5. Serve with some frozen fruit ice-cream and garnish with a sprig of fresh mint and a large strawberry split to sit on the side of the glass.

Banana Split

B L D

☺ ☺ ☹

10 minutes to make
Serves 4 adults

Ingredients

4 large ripe bananas
3 cups low-fat vanilla jello
1½ cups low-fat natural yogurt
8 teaspoons honey
2 dessertspoons raisins

Method

1. Peel then slice the bananas down the centre and place in 4 suitable dishes.
2. Pour the desired amount of yogurt and jello over them in a messy fashion.
3. Dribble honey over the dish and toss in raisins.
4. Serve with a cup of fat free hot chocolate made with non-fat milk.

Honey and Lemon Crêpes

B L D

20 minutes to make
Serves 4–6 adults

Ingredients
2 cups plain flour
4 cups non-fat milk
2 eggs
2 cups fresh seasonal fruit, roughly chopped
2 lemons
honey

Method
1. Mix flour, milk and eggs in a bowl until light and airy.
2. In a very hot non-stick pan, pour in enough mixture to form a crêpe the size of a salad plate.
3. When air bubbles appear on top of the crêpe and moisture has evaporated, carefully turn crêpe over.
4. After 30 seconds or so, slide crêpe out onto large plate.
5. Place fresh fruit into centre of crêpe, then roll into a loose tube.
6. Serve with honey and lemon.

Strawberries with a Balsamic Reduction

B L D

10 minutes to make
Serves 4 adults

Ingredients
3 cups fresh strawberries
1 ½ cup balsamic vinegar
¼ cup brown sugar
1 cup Greek non-fat yogurt with no added sugar

Method
1. Wash and drain the strawberries and place into four separate serving bowls or glasses.
2. Pour the balsamic vinegar into a saucepan and bring to a boil, followed by reducing the heat to a simmer.
3. When reduced halfway, add the brown sugar.
4. Simmer until it becomes syrupy and sticks to the back of a wooden spoon.
5. Drizzle balsamic reduction over strawberries.
6. Add a dollop of Greek yogurt and serve.

Snacks

- ★ Devilled Eggs

- ★ Greek Yogurt with Honey and Berries

- ★ Chicken Strips with Fresh Salsa

- ★ Mocha Protein Smoothie

- ★ Blueberry Protein Cakes

Devilled Eggs

B L D

 ☺ ☺ ☺

30 minutes to make
24 servings

Ingredients

12 hard-cooked eggs
½ cup fat free mayonnaise
2 teaspoon Dijon mustard
2 tablespoon green onions, finely chopped
1 tablespoon chives, finely chopped
Paprika

Method

1. Cut cooked eggs in half lengthwise.
2. Scoop out yolks and place them in a bowl.
3. Mash the egg yolks with a fork; add mayonnaise, mustard and green onions. Mix well.
4. Spoon yolk mixture into egg halves.
5. If you have a pastry bag with a star-shaped tip, you can pipe the yolks into the whites.
6. Top with chives.
7. Cover and refrigerate until ready to use.
8. Sprinkle with a little paprika before serving if you like.

Greek Yogurt with Honey and Berries

B L D

 ☺ ☺ ☺

15 minutes to make
12 servings

Ingredients
12 small 'shot' glasses
3 cups plain low fat Greek Yogurt
2 cups mixed berries chopped
1/2 cup honey
12 small sprigs fresh mint

Method
1. Set out 12 glasses.
2. Fill each glass with yogurt ¾ full.
3. Drizzle honey over the yogurt in each glass.
4. Add chopped berries to the top.
5. Garnish with a sprig of mint.
6. Refrigerate and serve chilled.

Chicken Strips with Fresh Salsa

B L D

  ☺

10 minutes to make
12 servings

Ingredients

5 large chicken breasts
4 ripe tomatoes, seeded and chopped
2 jalapeno peppers, seeded and chopped
1 medium onion, chopped
4 tablespoons fresh chopped cilantro
1 garlic clove, finely chopped
2 tablespoons fresh lime juice
salt and pepper to taste

Method

1. Cut the chicken into strips and grill on a barbeque or indoor grill and set aside.
2. If you've never chopped jalapenos or other hot peppers before, be sure to wear latex or other protective gloves.
3. Combine chopped ingredients in a bowl and, if you're not in a hurry, refrigerate for at least an hour to let the flavors mingle.
4. Serve the chicken strips on a platter with the salsa in a bowl with a serving spoon.

Mocha Protein Smoothie

B L D

2 minutes to make
Serves 1 adult

Ingredients
1 serving of protein powder
1 shot espresso coffee
1 teaspoon non-fat drinking chocolate
1 cup non-fat milk
1 cup water

Method
1. Using a container which will hold up to 3 cups of liquid, pour in the milk. [Make sure the milk is added first!]
2. Add the other ingredients.
3. Blend well.
4. Drink right away while chilled, or take with you in a container to drink throughout the day.

Blueberry Protein Cakes

B L D

15 minutes to make
makes 8 mini cakes

Ingredients

1 container fresh blueberries
2 cups whey protein concentrate
2 cups self-rising flour
2 eggs
2 cups non-fat milk

Method

1. In a small non-stick saucepan, lightly simmer the blueberries until soft.
2. Combine all ingredients in a large mixing bowl. The mixture should be of a pancake-like consistency.
3. Preheat a large non-stick frying pan.
4. Spoon in the mixture, four pancakes at a time. Be careful to flip them over before they burn.
5. When the other side has almost cooked through, remove quickly from the pan.
6. Serve right away. These go stale after half a day, so only make what you need.

Party Appetizers

★   Garlic King Shrimp

★   Cold Dip Platter

★   San Choy Bow

★   Pizzettas with Sun-dried Tomatoes

★   Salmon and Potato Croquettes

Garlic King Shrimp

B L D

10 minutes to make
Serves 8 adults

Ingredients

½ cup fat free chicken stock
4 teaspoons crushed garlic
1 teaspoon finely chopped parsley
1 teaspoon salt
40 large, fresh, uncooked jumbo shrimp, peeled and deveined
½ cup white wine
1 lemon
pepper to taste

Method

1. In a large non-stick frying pan, heat the stock, garlic, parsley and salt.
2. When the mixture is very hot, add the shrimp and white wine, stirring constantly.
3. The shrimp will be cooked in just a few minutes. They need to be served immediately with their sauce in a preheated dish with a wedge of lemon.

Cold Dip Platter

B L D
 ☺ ☺

10 minutes to make
Serves at least 8 adults

Ingredients
4 medium-sized carrots
3 celery stalks
8 medium-sized mushrooms
1 red pepper
1 green pepper
1 cup yellow squash
2 small tomatoes
handful of fresh snow peas
1 cup salsa
1½ cups low-fat ricotta cheese
¾ cup sweet mustard pickles
1½ cups apple sauce

Method
1. Wash all the vegetables and slice into finger-sized pieces.
2. Using a large, open platter, arrange the vegetables into their own section.
3. In the middle, place three small bowls containing the salsa, ricotta cheese mixed with sweet mustard pickles, and apple sauce.
4. Serve chilled and fresh.

San Choy Bow

B L D

20 minutes to make
Serves 8 adults

Ingredients
1½ pound very lean beef, minced
1 medium onion, diced
1 teaspoon garlic salt
2 cups small broccoli heads
2 cups small cauliflower heads
1 cup shredded carrot
1 cup shredded cabbage
1 teaspoon Chinese spices
pepper to taste
8 large, crisp, iceberg lettuce leaves

Method
1. In a hot, medium-sized non-stick frying pan, toss the beef, onion and garlic salt.
2. When cooked, add all the vegetables except the lettuce, and cover with a lid. Cook until vegetables are only just soft [should still be very firm].
3. Trim the large lettuce leaves so they resemble the shape of a bowl.
4. Spoon the warm mince mixture into the cold lettuce leaves, sprinkle with pepper, and serve immediately.

Pizzettas with Sun-dried Tomatoes

B L D

15 minutes to make
Serves 8 adults

Ingredients
1 long French breadstick, cut into 12 pieces
½ cup sun-dried tomatoes [not in oil]
chopped fresh basil
1 cup tomato purée
balsamic vinegar
salt and pepper to taste

Method
1. This recipe is very easy. Spread each slice of the French stick with tomato purée.
2. Sprinkle with a little fresh basil.
3. Top with some chopped sun-dried tomatoes.
4. Drizzle with a little balsamic vinegar and top with salt and pepper.
5. Grill until the sides of the pizzettas are golden brown and serve immediately.

Salmon and Potato Croquettes   B L D

25 minutes to make
Serves 8 adults

Ingredients

A little non-fat milk
6 medium large washed potatoes
1 large can salmon [as little oil as possible]
2 egg
1 large onion, finely chopped
2 teaspoons fat free chicken stock powder
3 large spring onion stalks, finely chopped
2 teaspoons pepper
½ teaspoon salt
4 tablespoons corn flour [a little extra if necessary]
2 tablespoons water
1 lemon wedges for garnish

Method

1. Boil potatoes in water with skin on. When cooked, mash with a little skim milk and put in mixing bowl.
2. Mix salmon, potatoes and remaining ingredients.
3. Take heaping teaspoons of mixture and roll in your hands in a croquette shape. Roll it in a little corn flour on a sheet of wax paper. Add enough corn flour so mixture is not too wet.
4. Place the salmon croquettes in a preheated pan.
5. When they have browned slightly on one side, turn them over, add a little water and place lid on the pan.
6. Watch the croquettes carefully. When they have browned, turn off the heat. Serve hot or cold with salad.

FYI

Concluding Thoughts

Parting words of encouragement.

Prioritize what matters and life will be amazing,
Body & Soul!

I read an amazing story about the importance of prioritizing our lives, so that we can live the life we imagine. The life we imagine starts with us making a decision that our future can be different; that it can be brighter. Remember to keep the main things the main things and enjoy the journey ahead!

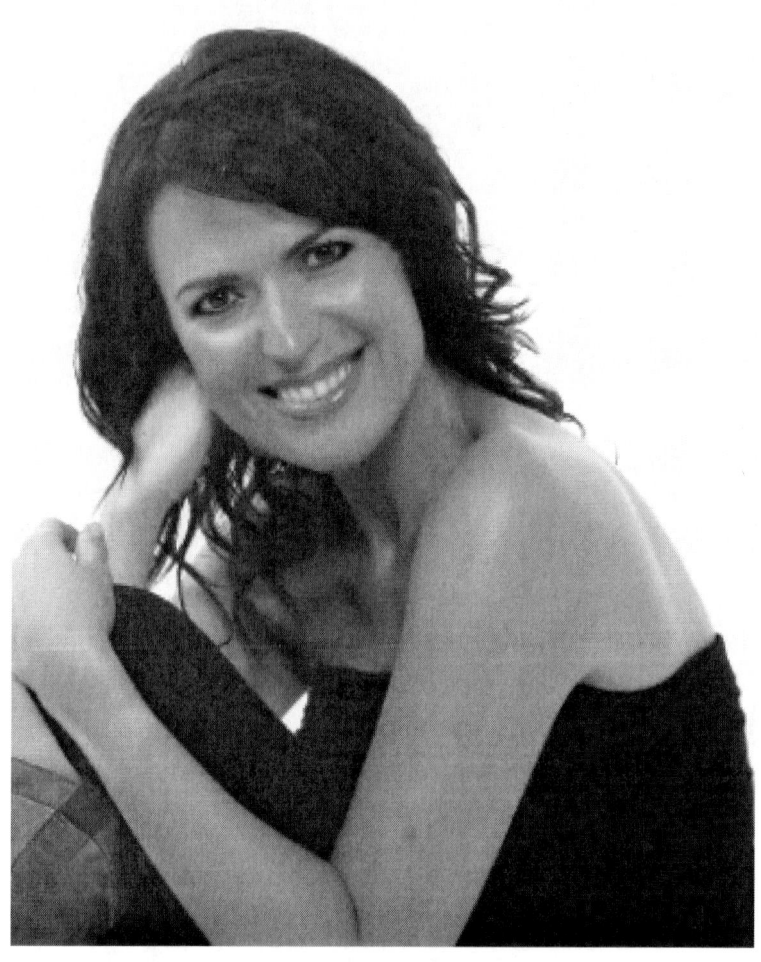

I love you!
I believe in you!
Thank you!

A philosophy professor stood before his class and had placed some items in front of him. When class began, without speaking, he picked up a large empty jar and proceeded to fill it with rocks, rocks about 2" in diameter. He then asked the students if the jar was full? They agreed that it was.

The professor then picked up a box of pebbles and poured them into the jar. He shook the jar lightly. The pebbles, of course, rolled into the open areas between the rocks. He then asked the student again if the jar was full. They agreed it was. The students laughed. The professor picked up a box of sand and poured it into the jar. Of course, the sand filled up everything else.

"Now," said the professor, "I want you to recognize that this is your life. The rocks are the important things - your family, your partner, your health, your children - anything that is so important to you that if it were lost, you would be nearly destroyed. The pebbles are the other things that matter - like your job, your house, your car. The sand is everything else. The small stuff."

"If you put the sand into the jar first, there is no room for the pebbles or the rocks. The same goes for your life. If you spend all your energy and time on the small stuff, you will never have room for the things that are important to you. Pay attention to the things that are critical to your well-being, body, soul and spirit. Pray to God. Read your Bible, Play with your children. Take time to get medical checkups. Take your partner out for date-night. There will always be time to go to work, clean the house, give a dinner party and fix the dishwasher."

"Take care of the rocks first - the things that really matter. Set your priorities. The rest is just sand."

Your Stories

Dear Dianne

Just a note to say thank you for this book! I'm thrilled to say that your eating plan has worked absolute wonders for me... There is now 30 pounds less of me! Very exciting and so easy! I remember being very discouraged before I read your book. I looked and felt incredibly fat. [I'm thirty-seven years old, but for my first twenty-six years, I looked like a stick. Ate whatever I wanted. Then came the beginnings of middle-age spread ... I thought that the spare tire was there to stay!]

I started your plan the day after I read your book, following it exactly. I've never eaten so much [quality] food in my life, yet the first 5 pounds literally fell off in the first week. That was encouraging. I weaned myself from high fat to low fat Breakfast is huge for me now! And thank God for those 'fat free' yoghurts.

By the way, a friend recently lost 30 pounds also using your book, and his Doctor was blown away! His triglyceride and cholesterol counts are within normal parameters already. He'd been told it would take three years.

Thank you!

Ian

Your Stories

Dear Dianne

Never before have I written to an author! I just had to on this occasion. I'm a self-confessed diet/health/fitness fanatic. I understand a lot about my body and how it works.

Well, I thought I did.

I knew what to do, and I ate as healthily as I knew how. Then I plateaued. Nothing would kick-start me. My problem area was my tummy and I was desperate to get rid of it. At thirty-five and after two Caesareans I knew it wouldn't be perfect, but I wanted it better than it was and I believed I could have it.

Then I saw your book ... and it immediately excited and inspired me, not only to change my eating habits but to source out another gym and have them design a new program for me. Time is something I don't have [like everyone else], so it's really important to get it all right.

Thank you! This makes more sense than anything I've read. I'm going to buy a copy for my mum [who's overweight] and I've been recommending it to all who'll listen — yes! It can't fail!

Denise

Your Stories

Dear Dianne

I've just finished reading your book! It was great, you did a great job, it's easy to understand and it makes sense...

I am 39 years old, 5'4" tall and started off weighing 190 pounds. I lost 10 pounds while on holiday a few weeks ago when I started your program.

Thank you!

Hi Dianne

I am so excited - I've now lost 16 pounds in 6 weeks! Thanks for the inspiration :)

Jenny

Dear Dianne

I just wanted to say that I really loved the book you wrote. Thank you very much for it. I have always been obsessed about my weight. I used to always think I was too fat and I started going on diets and not eating at all.

My friends have read your book too and they loved it as well. It's working and I can notice it.

Thanks again, and I hope to meet you one day.

Sonja

Your Stories

Hi Dianne

I just started week 7 and am 31 pounds down! I am absolutely loving it and feel fantastic! Your book has given me great understanding! Thank you so much for helping me.

Donna

Dianne

I really want to thank you for the blessing you have had on my life... I have battled with my weight for 10 years after the birth of my first little girl. You have given me the inspiration to claim my identity and make a change. Thank you!

Judith

Hey Dianne

Your book is sooo good!

For 4 years I have been yo-yo dieting......[by the way you look soooo gorgeous! A total inspiration!] I would lose 5 pounds then gain 5 pounds, etc., been doing this since the birth of my 3rd child. But now, I love the thought of commitment.....if you can lose 5 pounds....you can lose 10, etc!

Laura

The BESTSELLER revised and updated

fat free forever!

The Body Shaping Lifestyle

RESULTS
RESULTS
RESULTS

Dianne Wilson

After giving birth to twins in 1994, age 27

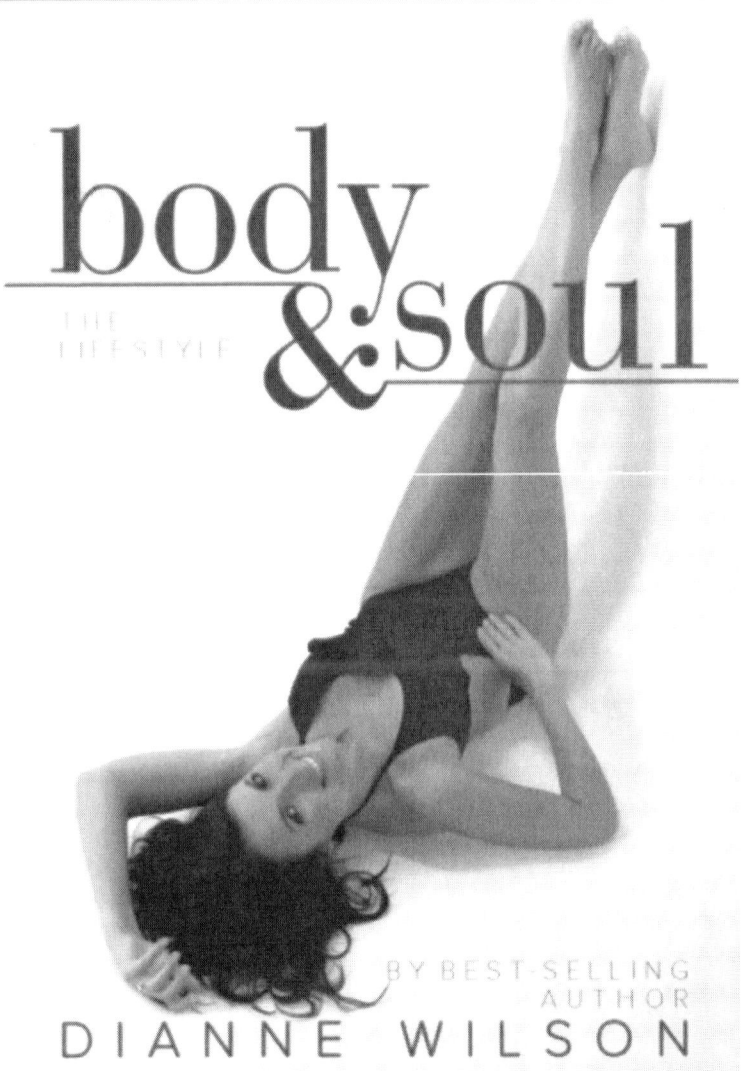

THE BESTSELLER REVISED & UPDATED

body
THE
LIFESTYLE
&soul

BY BEST-SELLING
AUTHOR
DIANNE WILSON

After giving birth to 4 babies, age 41

The night before I began this journey of
Body & Soul,
I opened a Thanksgiving bon-bon and inside
was a little piece of paper which reminded me
that God would be with me…
I tucked the little piece of paper away,
and now I pray that these words inspire you
as they inspired me.

*"No obstacles will stand in the way
of your success."*

God is with you!
GO FOR IT!